Ménière's Woman

when life gives you lemons ...

Julieann Wallace

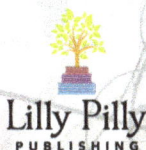

Lilly Pilly
PUBLISHING

This book was not created with or by AI. Forgive me for any errors. I will update the book as they are found.

Ménière's disease is a debilitating vestibular condition that causes vertigo, hearing loss, tinnitus, brain fog, fullness of the ear, balance difficulties. It is life changing. Any medical research in this book is supported by the URL of the research paper or publication or site.

MEDICAL DISCLAIMER:

Although the author has made every effort to ensure that the information in this book was correct at press time, the author does not assume and hereby disclaims any liability to any party for any loss, damage, or disruption caused by errors or omissions, whether such errors or omissions result from negligence, accident, or any other cause.

The information provided in this book is designed to support, not replace, the relationship that exists between a patient and his/her existing health care professionals. *** No medicinal content on this site, regardless of date, should ever be used as a substitute for direct medical advice from your doctor or other qualified clinician.

Book Cover design by Julieann Wallace Cover art 123RF: 180280314
1st Edition
ISBN: 978-0-6451581-9-9 (print book)
ISBN: 978-0-6480382-7-6 (eBook)

Dedicated to my *husband*, for being by my side in the incredibly low and dark Ménière's days, and for your patience as we searched for a treatment that would put some of the pieces of me back together again. Somehow, I think Humpty Dumpty understands.

Dedicated to my Ménière's sisters with love and understanding ~ take my hand. xx

be *kind*

to yourself.
It's the key to
healing and growing.

Ménière's Disease

Prosper Menière (18 June 1799 – 7 February 1862) was a French doctor who first identified a medical condition combining vertigo, hearing loss and tinnitus, which is now known as Menière's disease. It's a disorder of the inner ear.

Very briefly, Ménière's disease causes episodes of:
• vertigo (episodes of feeling like the world is spinning)
• tinnitus - ranging from mild to severe.
• a feeling of fullness or pressure in the ear.
• sudden falls without loss of consciousness (drop attacks) may be experienced by some people, or a sensation of being pushed sharply to the floor from behind.
• low-frequency hearing loss, which usually fluctuates in the beginning stages and becomes ore permanent in later stages, so that little or no hearing remains.
• a common and important symptom of MD is hypersensitivity to sounds, also known as hyperacusis.

Attacks may be characterized by periods of dormancy and exacerbation. After a severe attack, most people find that they are extremely exhausted and must sleep for several hours. People with Ménière's disease may suffer from psychological distress, high anxiety and depression. It is important to note that many people suffering from MD lead productive, near-normal lives, while others face greater challenges in coping. There is no cure for Ménière's disease - yet. But with advances in medicine and research, there is hope for a cure.

* **BPPV** - *Benign paroxysmal positional vertigo* is one of the most common causes of vertigo — the sudden sensation that you're spinning or that the inside of your head is spinning. BPPV causes brief episodes of mild to intense dizziness. It is usually triggered by specific changes in your head's position. BPPV can be resolved by the Epley Maneuver, or similar positional manoeuvres by your health professional.
* **PPPD** - *Persistent Postural-Perceptual Dizziness* are persistent sensations of rocking or swaying unsteadiness and/or dizziness without vertigo lasting 3 months or more.

About
Ménière's Woman

My shadow, Ménière's, has been with me for 29 years at the time of writing this book. Exactly half of my lifetime. It was a very difficult first ten years, where I would be debilitated for four hours or more at a time with horrendous violent vertigo at least forty times a year. Ménière's an absolute life changer. I developed a chronic fear of vertigo attacks, and PTSD, and so stopped shopping by myself, socialising, driving, and teaching. Everyday I kept a diary of what I ate or drank, where I had been and what I had done, to see if I could find the trigger for my attacks.

I woke at daybreak, early one day in January 2024, with the words "Ménière's Man" in my mind. And then I thought of all the books written by men with Ménière's disease, and decided it was time to have a Ménière's book written by a woman! Researchers have uncovered countless ways in which women's and men's bodies react differently to the same diseases, due to our hormones. There is A LOT that female bodies to go through during a hormonal cycle, a stark contrast to the experience of the male body.

It is my hope that this book can help you. I have put countless hours into research and reading anecdotal stories by women, and my own experience. Some suggestions in this book may help you. Trial and error is the ball game of Ménière's disease, as you know. By keeping a track of your daily living with Ménière's, you may find a pattern that will help you with your battle against it. As you are using the period journal tracker, highlight symptoms, add symptoms, add notes about what you are experiencing, or any new symptoms, plus vertigo length and severity. And because this is your book, add your own stamp and style. I have left blank pages for your to glue/tape in clippings, inspirational verses or images that speak to you in some way, or write them in. Be creative. Be *you*.

It is my forever hope and prayer, that a cure or successful treatments are found.

Julieann xo

Contents

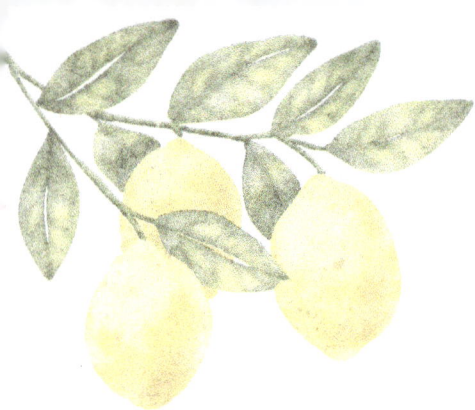

Lemons

They say when life gives you lemons, make lemonade.

"They" obviously don't have Ménière's disease, or any other incurable, debilitating, life changing disease for that matter. If they did, they *would* say, 'I'm sorry about your diagnosis. I hope a cure comes soon. Let me know if you ever need help with anything.'

I want to say that I am sorry that you have Ménière's disease. I wouldn't wish it on my worst enemy. I have had it since I was twenty-nine, have had three kids, gone through perimenopause and menopause.

I woke at 5am one morning in early January, 2024, with the words *Ménière's Man* stuck in my head. It's a book written about Ménière's disease, by a man. I've never read it. But I know that people are thankful for the information inside it. Then I thought, where are the Ménière's books written by women?

How about WOMénière's? WO<u>ménière's</u>? woMénière's?

Sure, you may be able to glean lots of interesting information from books written by men, but let's face it, they don't deal with holding the responsibility of keeping the household going like women do (mostly) – groceries, cooking, cleaning, childcare (if you do have a partner who helps you with that, you are truly blessed!).

Men don't deal with menstruation and everything that entails.

Men don't have babies.

Men don't go through perimenopause and menopause.

Men don't have the fluctuations with hormones like women do.

So, this book is for us. Ménière's Woman.

On the pages you'll find tips, hints, research, personal anecdotes, secret women's business, pregnancy, motherhood, grand-motherhood, understanding, inspiration and ... lemon recipes.

And for those with faith, I have included a place for that as well.

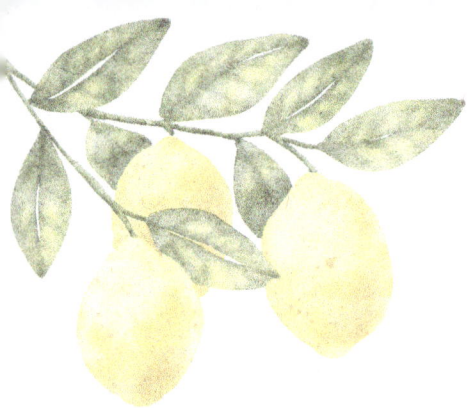

My story

'I'm sorry. There is no cure.'
I die a little inside each time I hear someone with Ménière's disease pleading for help, saying they can't do it anymore, and when I hear the call-out for prayer for someone who is suicidal from the insidious, incurable Ménière's disease ... I've been there.

I know exactly how it feels.

I wish I had a magic wand to heal every one of us. Right now.

Let me tell you the short story version of my journey.

1995 ...

'I'm sorry. There is no cure.'

'No cure?'

'No ... no cure. No cause. But you're not going to die from it.' My ear specialist eyed me with caution. The bitterness of my diagnosis after five hours of testing was painful to acknowledge.

'Let's wait and see how your symptoms go,' he said.

I stepped out of the ENT's office, trailed by a very dark shadow: Ménière's disease. It was so large it cast a darkness over me like a heavy storm cloud, ready to erupt into the strong spiralling wind of a cyclone at any moment.

I knew the symptoms of my diagnosis well.

I lived them with every breath that I took, mixed with fear and anxiety: aural fullness, hearing loss, tinnitus, and vertigo – the abhorrent violent vertigo – a life destroyer.

I felt like I was given a prison sentence.

Where was the key to escape from Ménière's disease?

Wait and see how my symptoms go?

Why?

'You could have a mild form of Ménière's disease that has little impact on your life, or it could go into remission,' he had said.

But mine didn't.

Rewind
My first symptom – 1994

At the age of 28 I had a blocked left ear, like I had been swimming. It felt full.

Except, I hadn't been swimming. It was winter.

I tried swimmers ear drops to clear that blocked feeling, numerous times, which didn't help, and then put up with it, assuming it would correct itself.

Except it didn't.

At the age of 29, I finally went to my doctor. She looked in my ear with her otoscope. Picture perfect for an ear canal by all accounts. She handed me a referral to an ear, throat and nose doctor (ENT).

I waited three months for my appointment, my ear still feeling full. After initial greetings, my ENT asked questions to create a profile of me.

Never smoked.

Not a drinker.

Healthy diet.

Active.

Healthy body.

He got out his tuning fork and struck it against his knee, producing a pure tone. I smiled inside, due to my familiarity of the tuning fork which I used when studying music at university. He placed the vibrating tuning fork on the mid-line of the forehead, the bridge of my nose, and chin, equidistant from both ears. These vibrations conducted through the skull to reach the cochlea.

My ENT asked questions like, 'Is the sound louder in your right ear, left ear, or the middle?' It was louder in my right ear.

The Weber test has been mainly used to establish a diagnosis in patients with unilateral hearing loss to distinguish between conductive and sensorineural hearing loss. It is a useful, quick, and simple screening test for evaluating hearing loss. The test can detect unilateral conductive and sensorineural hearing loss.

With the absence of any other symptoms, my ENT ordered an MRI, to eliminate inner ear problems, due to injury or disease, or tumours.

The MRI came back clear. Which then lead to the scenario of let's wait and see what other symptoms you have. I asked what he was looking for, and he said, 'Ménière's disease of Multiple Sclerosis.'

It was a waiting game.

Rewind
Prior to my first symptom – early 1994

Bell's Palsy

The new school year was a week away. I was keen, excited and raring to go to meet my new students. While grocery shopping with my husband, I noticed that the left half of my tongue felt numb. Heart rate up.

We continued shopping, my telling myself that I was most probably imaging it.

After a little while longer, I noticed the left side of my face starting to tingle. Heart rate up again.

We continued shopping. I must have been imagining it.

At home that afternoon, I couldn't close my left eye. The left side of my mouth wouldn't move. Heart rate up and stayed there.

We went to emergency at the hospital. The first test there was for a stroke. And a blood test. I had neither of those, and was given the diagnosis of Bell's Palsy based on my set of symptoms. I was given oral steroids and sent on my way.

My Bell's Palsy lasted two weeks. It was most definitely a big scare. What set it off? Was it the hair dressing appointment just prior to it, where my neck was really uncomfortable at the wash basin? What is a virus? Was it something I had done?

I never got any answers.

Rewind
The year I was 16

Sport was my life. I was a fast runner and excelled at school in sport. I played all the sports offered to me, often invited to because of my natural skill. Sport made me happy. Happier. Happiest.

By the time I reached sixteen, I was playing at the highest level at the softball club I had been a playing at since I was twelve. They pulled me out of under 16s to the highest women's competition. All were seasoned softball players. Accurate, fast-paced lethal throwers, pitchers, batters, base runners. Commitment and passion for the game. And training.

One night at training, we were standing in a line, two arms-space apart, with a partner opposite us. Accurate, fast-paced lethal throwers, the ball hurtling fast toward partners. The sound of the ? as the ball was caught in the glove.

My partner threw a ball, a little way side. I stretched out to catch it but it hit the end of my glove and landed on the ground between me and the person to my right. I bent over to pick it up and

WHACK!!!

I copped a lethal softball (which is rock hard by the way – I don't know why they call it soft ball because the ball is anything but soft) on the side of my face, directly in front of my ear on the cheek bone. Had it been higher on my head, on my temple, I probably wouldn't be writing this book.

Gasps sounded and training stopped. The coach came over to me and put his hand on my shoulder. 'Are you alright?'

I placed my hand over the side of my face, on the side of my jaw and opened and closed my jaw. It worked okay. All my teeth were still there. There was a little bit of pain, but not a lot. He was satisfied with that. We went back to training.

Mum picked me up from training and I told her I got hit in the side of the head. 'Are you okay?'

'Yes,' I said.

And that was that. No doctor visit. No hospital visit or x-ray. No check for concussion or other head trauma.

I went to school the next day like nothing had happened. In front of my ear on the bone was a little sore but not too bad. There was no bruising.

And the injury was long forgotten. Like it never happened.

Did the brute force of the impact damage my inner ear?

Did it put my jaw alignment out?

Did it affect the alignment of my neck?

I did discover, at the age of 54 that I was missing the cartilage disc of my left temporomandibular joint (TMJ), most probably caused by the impact trauma when I was 16. Did I have a clicking jaw? Absolutely. Most of my life. But when I had my dentist check for that issue, he didn't find any misalignment.

Return
to 1995 …

Waiting for symptoms. My ear remained feeling blocked, and nothing I could do would change that. It wasn't Eustachian Tube Dysfunction that caused it. It just was.

September 1995 …

I was pregnant. After trying to have a baby for years. Excited and scared. No Internet back then to Google pregnancy. Only a book like 'What to Expect When You Are Expecting', and information from the doctor and friends who had been through pregnancy, and the table discussions amongst pregnant teachers at school, and horror pregnancy and birthing stories. Women will understand that perfectly.

Curiously, my left ear felt clear for the first time since that symptom began.

Was it hormonal changes in my body?

September 1996

My baby is four months old. Adorable. Loved. Cherished.

It's Saturday. My husband is home.

And the room spins uncontrollably. Terribly fast. I can't stop it. It makes me nauseous. I can't close my eyes. All I can do is stare at one flower on the wallpaper to try to gain some sort of control. This is hell.

After two hours I sit up in bed. Shell-shocked. What was that? I'm terrified. I'm crying. I'm shattered. I'm scared it will happen again.

My husband drives me to my doctor. She gives me Stemetil for the nausea, and another referral to see my ENT.

My ENT orders tests to be conducted at a hospital. Five hours of tests.

- Hearing test
- Pure Tone Audiometry
- Head Impulse Test
- Electrocochleography
- Vestibular evoked myogenic potentials (VEMP) testing
- Caloric stimulation

And then he finally he gives my set of symptoms a name.

'You have Ménière's disease. It's mostly men over the age of fifty who have it.'

My symptoms started at twenty-eight, with the ear fullness.

'I'm sorry. There is no cure,' he says.

After the appointment, I walked out, stunned, with a script for a diuretic, and a warning to stay away from salt—which we never added to our food, ever.

Your story

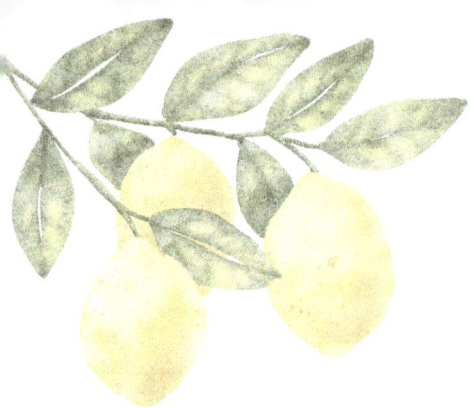

Dear Me,

One day, just like that ...

I'll re-discover my *light*.
I'll find my *strengths*.
I'll embrace my inner *warrior*.
I'll snatch my *power* back.

And the whole game will change.

Love, Me

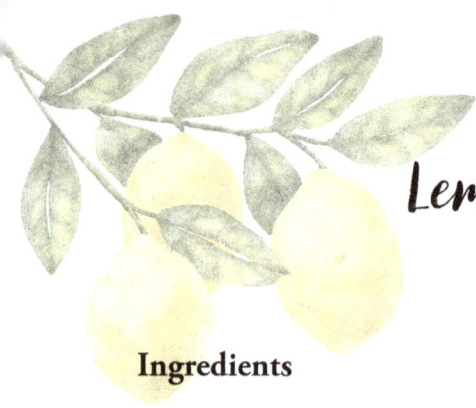

Lemonade

Ingredients

1 cup sugar (can reduce to 3/4 cup)
1 cup water (for the simple syrup)
1 cup freshly squeezed lemon juice
2 to 3 cups cold water, to dilute

Directions

1. *Lemons*
Juice your lemons. 4 to 6 of them should be enough for
1 cup of juice - depending on the size of the lemons.

2. *Simple syrup*
With the sugar and water in a small saucepan, bring it
to a simmer. Make sure your stir so that the sugar
dissolves completely. Remove the syrup from the heat.

3. *Create the lemonade*
Pour the juice and syrup sugar water into a pitcher.
You can add two to three cups of cold water if you would like
it to be more diluted (remember that if you add ice, it will
melt and naturally dilute the lemonade).
Too sweet? Add a little more lemon juice to it.

4. *Chill and serve.*
Refrigerate 30 to 40 minutes.

Serve with ice and sliced lemons.

Notes (thoughts, photos, tweaks to recipe)

Ménière's Disease

Ménière's disease. 0.02% of people around the world have it.

Welcome to the club that no one wants to be a part of.

No cause. No cure. This landscape is changing I believe. I'll talk more about that in research.

From my now twenty-nine years of Ménière's experience, I know that Ménière's disease is an absolute life changer. And not for the better. My life certainly changed. The change in my life and myself is so marked that I divide my life into before Ménière's disease, and after.

From my twenty-nine years of Ménière's experience, I need to ask you a question. Are you certain you have Ménière's disease? Have you been officially diagnosed? If not, get a diagnosis. What if, what you have can be fixed?

Before Ménière's Disease

Before Ménière's, sport was my passion, and music and art. I was a high-achiever in everything I did. Teaching was the career I chose and loved it with all my heart. I was that teacher who did the '40-Hour Famine' with students each year and won an award for it. I did 'Jump Rope for Heart' every year with the students, raising money for The Heart Foundation. I ran Scripture Union at lunchtimes, and Skipping Club before school. I was that teacher who always had the other teachers' children in my classes, by request.

I was a 'what'. I was known by my what. Over my teaching career I received two nominations for the National Excellence in Teaching Awards for my 'what'.

But then the unpredictable violent, debilitating vertigo of Ménière's hit. At least forty times a year. I was incapacitated for three or four hours each time, spinning at an impossible speed, staring at the wall for the entire time trying to cope with what my body was going through, vomiting until the only thing that came up was froth. I was a frequent flyer at emergency at the hospital for re-hydration, where I had to educate the doctors and nurses on my incurable disease they had no knowledge of. How many times had I been told that I was hyperventilating, or that it was "all in my head".

I pray that you never experience vertigo like I had.

Eventually, Ménière's took away what I loved to do. I could no longer participate in sport. Music was too loud, even though I was going deaf, due to the hyperacusis. Art went by the wayside. I couldn't teach. My confidence was stolen. I was no longer independent. I couldn't socialise anymore because of my hearing and the unpredictability of a vertigo attack. My food choices were severely limited. Ice was on the menu on some days. I was underweight. I lived every conscious moment in fear of an incapacitating vertigo attack. I would even wake in the middle of the night spinning for hours on end.

I became a prisoner in my own home. My own body. My own mind. Every day was like a battlefield, and the world became very dark.

What was the point of living a life like this?

Each time that I lay staring at the wall, spinning, wherever I was, even the floor in the toilet for four hours because I couldn't be moved during the vertigo, I had no more 'what'.

It was just me. With nothing. Like a brain with awareness and a decommissioned body experiencing the internal lie that I was spinning, and yet in reality, my physical body wasn't. I was capable of absolutely nothing. I felt like a nothing. I was a nothing.

I could move my arms and legs, but I couldn't move my head. If I did, it was catastrophic. The spinning was impossibly more terrifying. So, I did the only thing I could—I stared at one spot on a wall for three to four hours, wherever I was, spinning, exhausted from the spinning, the nausea, the vomiting. The only thing left I had was my mind.

Me and my mind. *Alone.* Experiencing a philosophical existential crisis way before it became a thing.

Successful Ménière's treatments or cures come soon, I pray.

If you are reading this book, it's because you or someone you know has Ménière's disease, so you will be familiar with the symptoms. If it is someone you know who has Ménière's, I want to thank you from the bottom of my heart for trying to understand Ménière's disease to help your partner, parent, sister, aunt, cousin or friend.

<u>Basic</u> Symptoms of Ménière's Disease

Hearing loss
Spontaneous, violent vertigo
Nausea
Vomiting
Ear fullness and sometimes pain
Tinnitus
Hearing loss
Deafness
Nystagmus
Extreme fatigue
Mental disorientation at times
Imbalance
Mood swings
Hyperacusis
Anxiety
Depression
+ *more*

After return visits to my ENT, I was given a diuretic and Stemetil. That was it. And that was all they had in 1996. End of story.

But was it?

When you are in the throes of debilitating vertigo, it's hard to see that it will ever get better. But it will. Ménière's is defined in four stages. The finish line is getting closer with each attack. In hindsight, stopping the MD beast at *stage one* is the ultimate target. Be proactive. Early in the disease. That was a choice I never had. You do.

Stages of Ménière's disease

I often find it comforting that Ménière's disease has stages. To me, it gives me a timeline of how long the Ménière's monster will keep sending me into a spin, and that there will be a definite end to the debilitating attacks. Seeing that finish line is encouraging and fills me with hope, when at times there seems like none. What we want to do though, to minimise damage, is to stop attacks.

Stage One
Sudden, unpredictable vertigo.
Hearing loss and tinnitus that comes and goes
Hearing and full sensation returns between attacks.

Stage Two
Vertigo attacks less severe
Hearing loss and damage develops. Tinnitus becomes worse
Periods of dormancy

Stage Three
Less frequent vertigo
Hearing loss becomes profound and tinnitus loud
Balance is affected

Burnout
No vertigo
Profound hearing loss. Multiple noises of tinnitus
Ear fullness remains
Balance affected

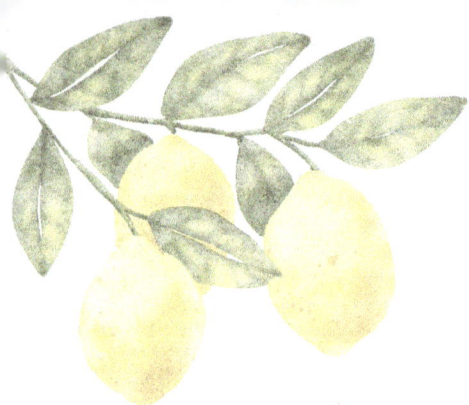

Dear Me,

Each morning when the *sun* greets
me, and the *birdsong* welcomes
the new day, I'm reminded that today
is a *new day*, to leave yesterday in
the past, and to *celebrate* my
wins, no matter how small. I am not
Ménière's disease, and Ménière's disease
is not me. And, my *good days*
far outnumber my bad days.

Love, Me

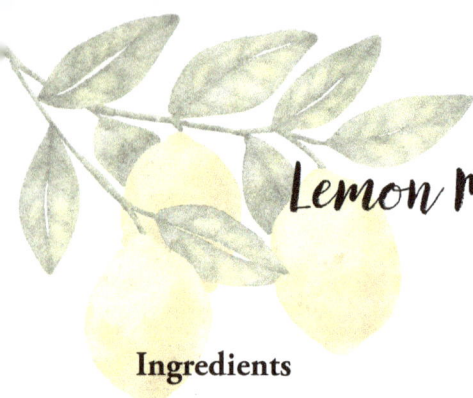

Lemon Meringue Pie

Ingredients

Filling
1 cup white sugar
2 tablespoons self-raising flour
3 tablespoons cornstarch
¼ teaspoon salt
1 ½ cups water
2 lemons, juiced and zested
2 tablespoons butter
4 egg yolks, beaten
1 baked pie crust

Meringue
4 egg whites
1/2 cup white sugar

Directions
Preheat the oven to 325ºF / 162º C.

To make the filling
1. Whisk 1 cup sugar, flour, cornstarch, and salt together
in a medium saucepan; stir in water, lemon juice, and
lemon zest. Cook over medium-high heat, stirring frequently,
until mixture comes to a boil. Stir in butter.

2. Place egg yolks in a small bowl and gradually whisk in 1/2 cup
of hot sugar mixture.
Whisk egg yolk mixture back into remaining sugar mixture.

Bring to a boil and continue to cook while stirring constantly until thick.

Remove from heat; pour filling into baked pastry shell.

To make the meringue

1. Beat egg whites in a glass, metal, or ceramic bowl with an electric mixer until foamy.

Gradually add sugar, continuing to beat until stiff peaks form.

Spread meringue over pie filling, sealing the edges at the crust.

2. Bake in preheated oven until meringue is golden brown, about 20 to 25 minutes.

Notes (thoughts, photos, tweaks to recipe)

Medications and Treatments

In 2004, nine years after my Ménière's started, I made a conscious decision to have my balance cells destroyed. I couldn't do the horrendous, unpredictable, debilitating, violent, torturous, insane, vertiginous spinning and nausea and vomiting and staring at one focus spot on the wall for the entire three-four hours anymore.

I was more than done. I didn't want to be here anymore. So when my ENT offered to inject gentamicin into my middle ear to kill off the balance cells, halting the vertigo, I didn't think twice.

Was the gentamicin my first port of call? Absolutely not. I had already had Ménière's disease for nine years and tried:

* Low salt diet
* Caffeine elimination
* Diet elimination
* Stemetil
* Diuretic
* Serc
* Sound therapy
* Acupuncture
* Herbal supplements
* Anti-viral - Acyclovir
* Prednisone
* Grommet

ENT wisdom … Least invasive treatments to most invasive. Our plan was to work through the list until we found something that worked for me, trying to preserve my hearing as much as we could.

Julieann wisdom … When deciding on a treatment, not only do you have to look at the physical side like a doctor, but also the emotional/mental side – how are you coping emotionally? Mentally? Psychologically? Socially? Depression? The best decisions are made with discussions with your medical carers and people who care about you e.g. partner, family, close friends. In the end, your call.

Gentamicin was next for me. If that didn't work, I was going to have a Vestibular Nerve Section. Thankfully, the gentamicin worked - an answered prayer. One full strength of Gentamicin injected in through my grommet into my inner ear, with some bicarbonate of soda and sterile water mixed with it to make it penetrate better. The procedure took place at my ENT's procedure room in the city. Before injecting the gentamicin, he spoke to Professor Bill Gibson, the MD guru, in Sydney. I laid on my right side while he injected the concoction in through my grommet in my left ear.

'Isn't that hurting?' he had asked me as he infused the mixture into my middle ear.

'Yes,' I had said, 'but I am envisaging it destroying the Ménière's in my middle ear. It's a mind visualisation technique I taught myself when I was young, when I had growing pains in my knees.'

I remained on my right side, left ear facing the ceiling for 20 minutes after the procedure, then went home, where I went to bed and rolled onto my right side to keep my left ear up. I slept for two hours.

The next day I had bouncy vision when I walked. It has a term – oscillopsia. Oscillopsia is a vision problem in which objects seem to jump, jiggle, or vibrate when they're actually still. It stems from a problem with the alignment of your eyes, or with the systems in your brain and inner ears that control your body alignment and balance. It was a side effect of having my balance cells destroyed. It was a good sign that the gentamicin was working, my ENT had said.

Three weeks later I was back teaching full-time, learning to trust that I wouldn't have anymore vertigo attacks. Since 2004, I have been vertigo free. So thankful for God's mercy and grace.

Choosing to destroy my balance cells to stop the vertigo was not a hard decision for me. Ménière's disease had total control of my life, and I wanted it back. There was a risk of losing all of my hearing, but that was a preferred choice compared to continual suffering through the torturous vertigo. The gentamicin stopped the vertigo. I gained quality of my life again – socialising, working, independence, driving, and slowly became more confident. I lost a little of my hearing, but not a lot.

If my vertigo returned, would I do it again? Yes. But that is also dependent on what new solutions for vertigo are around in the future.

When I joined global Ménière's groups, years later, I discovered that others who had this procedure done were having balance therapy. I was shocked that there was even a thing called balance therapy. When I had my procedure done in 2004, balance therapy/rehabilitation didn't exist where I lived. I had to relearn to walk again, finding my new balance, learning my limitations as I went. No help.

On the right page, I have created a list of prescription medications and alternative treatments that I have researched in medical studies and papers, on social media Ménière's group pages, and from my own experience.

There are many different names for the same drug around the world, so ensure you Google the medication name, and add "other names", to your search to see what they are commonly called in the country you live in, and absolutely **engage your doctor/specialist if you are considering any of the treatments, as some may not be suitable for you.** There's space for you to add your own treatments.

Some of the medications may not be available, depending on what year you are reading this book, and more may become available in the future that aren't listed here. Keep an eye out for new medications that come. You can record other medications here.

***The information provided in this book is designed to support, not replace, the relationship that exists between a patient and his/her existing health care professionals. The medications mentioned in this book must only be taken under the supervision of your medical health carer.**

Ménière's Disease

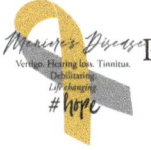

Possible treatments/medications checklist *Please note* - this is simply a list so you are **aware** of what medications/treatments may be available. **Always consult your doctor.**

Treatment/Medication	Effective	Treatment/Medication	Effective
Limit caffeine		Verapamil	
Limit alcohol		Nimodipine	
Limit tobacco		Cinnarizine	
Limit chocolate		Flunarizine	
Limit MSG		Diazepam	
Limit salt		Prednisone	
Limit sugars		Immune suppressants	
Dairy/lactose		Scopolamine patch	
Wheat/gluten		Cognitive Behaviour Therapy	
Cervical Alignment		Relaxation Techniques	
Acupuncture		John of Ohio Plan	
Diuretics		Urea	
Antiviral - e.g. Acyclovir		Medical Marijuana	
Prochlorperazine		Migraine medications	
Betahistine		Methotrexate (rarely)	
Meclizine		Enbrel (injectable drug)	
Lorazepam		Humira (injectable)	
Promethazine		Steroid ear injections	
Ondansetron (nausea)		Grommet	
Benzodiazepines		Dexamethasone	
Anti-depressants		Endolymphatic sac duct blocking (EDB)	
Anti-anxiety		Gentamicin	
TMJ		Endolymphatic Sac Decompression	
Dramamine			
Diphenhydramine		Vestibular Nerve Section	
Calcium Channel Blockers		Labyrinthectomy	
Prescription nasal sprays			
Eustachian tube dysfunction			

Natural Supplements, Alternative Treatments

As to diseases, make a habit of two things - to help, or at least, to do no harm - Hippocrates

Ménière's disease is frustrating.

Some prescription medicines work for some, but not others. Prescription medicine did not work for me. Alternative treatments didn't work for me as I tried to slay the Ménière's beast with my sword of knowledge and research and trialling of integrative medicines. I believe that it comes down to the cause of our Meniere's, which researchers agree, there is no one cause of Meniere's, and that's why finding successful treatment is so frustrating.

I'll talk more in depth about alternative treatments and supplements on page 182.

***Always check with your doctor or pharmacist that the supplements don't interact with other medications you take.**

During my Ménière's journey, particularly from 1999 onwards, I was frustrated, emotionally hurting and desperate to find my trigger for vertigo attacks. I kept daily notes of everything I ate and did to find patterns so I could change my diet, stress levels or lifestyle. This journal I created may help you (doctors love it because it shows what is happening in the lead up to a vertigo attack).

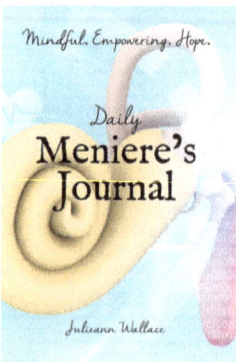

Ménière's Treatment Hope

Waiting for successful treatments seems to take forever. The trouble with Ménière's treatments, and other illness treatments, is not that there isn't anyone researching and creating treatments, it's that, once the researchers believe that have found a suitable treatment, they have to rigorously test the treatment, which then needs stringent medical testing and double blind trials.

The strict safety protocols of a drug is a key reason why the process of drug development takes time. There are numerous studies that regulators require in determining if a drug is safe enough to be dosed in humans—and these safety studies continue throughout clinical trials and the drug's life cycle.

There are many Ménière's treatment trials ongoing, globally, but I decided not to list them in this book because of the ever changing landscape of Ménière's trials and outcomes. For instance, Otonomy, a biotech company, collapsed after a phase 3 clinical trial of Otividex for Ménière's disease because it missed its primary endpoint.

If you are interested to read about Ménière's treatment trails, you can research it on the Internet. Be careful to check the year the trials happened, because you will still see trials and treatments listed that happened a long time ago, and nothing came of them.

In 2023, I was in a Teams meeting with a Ménière's researcher in Australia, and the question was asked about why researchers don't declare to the public what they are working. He said the reason was that they don't want to give false hope.

So don't be surprised when suddenly a successful treatments pop up catching you unawares. The highly regarded researcher also said that there won't be just one treatment that works for everyone, there will be many treatments, because they know that Ménière's develops due to a number of causes.

But rest assured that research is ongoing all over the world, as well as Ménière's Symposiums and Conferences where the researchers come together to share their findings. If you Google Ménière's Symposiums and Conferences, you will find when they are happening ,and where they are happening around the world.

Whilst researching Ménière's treatments online, beware:

- Date of the trial

How long ago was it?

Did anything ever become of the drug in the trial?

Was it effective or not?

- Is the trial recent?

A cure or effective treatment for Ménière's *will* come. Having had Ménière's since 1995, I have seen a ridiculous amount of information unfold and discoveries made about it. And with current technology, and the further development of technology, it will allow researchers to go further than they ever have, and the use of nanotechnology and nanobots will allow entry into the inner ear giving answers for questions long asked.

At the time of writing this book (2024), Ménière's researchers in Australia are about to trial an implantable device that will allow us to turn off the vertigo and restore our balance.

But right now, you need to have your own plan to look after you.

Seek wisdom from your doctor/specialist, or if your specialist or doctor say there is nothing they can do, find one who is willing to journey with you to find solutions.

Delve deeper and ask questions in Ménière's social media groups. You will find a wealth of experience and information there, and doctors and specialists who are supportive.

Remember, *least invasive to most invasive.*

However, if you are in a very dark place, mentally, it may be time to fast track to a more invasive treatment. In hindsight, had I have known how bad my Ménière's was going to be and its effect on my whole person, as well as limiting life experiences of my three children because I couldn't go out anywhere with them by myself, I should have chosen the Gentamicin treatment sooner.

For the next pages, I will categorize treatments from least invasive to most invasive. I'll also give you detailed information about the treatments I have researched online at:

brainfoundation.org.au/disorders/menieres-disease
mayoclinic.org/diseases-conditions/menieres-disease
nidcd.nih.gov/health/menieres-disease
my.clevelandclinic.org/health/diseases/15167-menieres-disease
menieres.org.uk
vestibular.org (VEDA)

Least Invasive

Medicines for vertigo that *may* make a vertigo attack less severe. Please be aware that the medications help some people, but not others. Ménière's loves us like that!
** You will find it helpful to find the medication names online for those listed here.

- Motion sickness medicines such as meclizine or diazepam may lessen the spinning feeling and help control nausea and vomiting.
- Anti-nausea medicines such as promethazine might control nausea and vomiting during a vertigo attack.
- Diuretics lower how much fluid is in the body, which may lower the amount of extra fluid in the inner ear.
- Betahistine (Serc) ease vertigo symptoms by improving blood flow to the inner ear.

Lifestyle Changes

Lifestyle changes are things that you consciously choose to change to enable a better quality of life. If I was making lifestyle changes, I wouldn't do all of this changes at the same time, as you won't know what has helped you. But the choice is up to you, as well.

- *Eat more frequent but smaller meals:* Evenly distributing meals throughout the day helps regulate body fluids. Rather than eating three large meals a day, try six smaller ones.
- *Drink water regularly,* and take particular care to hydrate regularly during hot weather and intense exercise.
- Tyramine, an amino acid found in a range of foods, including chicken liver, smoked meats, red wine, ripe cheeses, nuts, and yogurts *may* trigger migraine, and Ménière's symptoms.
- *Low salt.* Limit sodium to 1200-1500mg a day. This *may* help control Ménière's disease symptoms. The less salt consumed, the less fluid your body will retain. Avoid adding salt to meals and cut out most junk foods, as these are often high in added salt. Please note, that cutting out salt entirely will lead to low sodium levels, and can lead to muscle cramps, nausea, vomiting and dizziness. Eventually, lack of salt can lead to shock, coma and death.
- *Avoid* alcohol, caffeine and nicotine, which can also change the fluid in the inner ear.
- *Stress and anxiety.* Doctors are unsure whether stress and anxiety cause symptoms, or whether Ménière's leads to stress and anxiety. However, managing your stress and anxiety help reduce symptoms or intensity of symptoms.
- *Additional rest.* Being overtired may trigger symptoms.
- *Rehabilitation.* Vestibular rehabilitation therapy might improve your balance if you have balance problems between vertigo attacks. You do exercises and activities to help your body and brain regain the ability to process balance.
- *Hearing technology.* Ménière's is sneaky. It steals your hearing bit by bit, and sometimes you are unaware of how much hearing you have lost until it is really obvious. Or, you are in denial about your hearing loss not wanting to acknowledge it. Or, you think you are coping well will your hearing loss ... until you try a hearing aid and discover what a massive difference it makes to your life, even masking the tinnitus sometimes. Wearing a hearing aid in the ear Ménière's ear might improve your hearing (YAY!). So make sure you

have your hearing checked regularly by an audiologist to talk about the best hearing aids for you.

• *Cochlear implant.* When a hearing aid no longer enables you to hear (like me), a cochlear implant will enable your hearing again. This hearing technology can be a life changer. I can not speak highly enough of it and how my life is so much better!

More Invasive Treatments

• *Grommet* - inserted into the eardrum to allow air into the middle ear space because it is connected at the back of the nose to the Eustachian tube. It is thought that it is possible that the pressure in the two systems might be different and grommets will allow that pressure to equalise.

Middle ear injections

Middle ear injections are absorbed in the middle ear and may help vertigo symptoms improve, or get better. This treatment is done in your health carer's office. Injections can include:

• *Gentamicin* is an antibiotic that's toxic to your inner ear. It works by damaging the part of your inner ear that's causing the vertigo. Your healthy ear then takes on the job for balance. There may be a risk of further hearing loss. This is what I had done in 2004.

• *Steroids* such as dexamethasone may help control vertigo attacks. Dexamethasone may not work as well as gentamicin. But it's less likely to cause further hearing loss.

Surgery

If vertigo attacks are severe and absolutely debilitating, or if your mental health is at risk and other treatments don't help, surgery might be an option for you.

- *Endolymphatic sac surgery* helps control inner ear fluid levels. This procedure relieves pressure around the endolymphatic sac, which *can* improve fluid levels. A discussion about the success rates of this procedure with your ear specialist would be recommended.
- *Labyrinthectomy.* The surgeon removes the parts of your ear causing vertigo, which causes complete hearing loss in that ear. This allows your healthy ear to be in charge of sending information about balance and hearing to your brain. Specialists only suggest this procedure if you have poor hearing or total hearing loss in your Ménière's ear.
- *Vestibular nerve section* involves cutting the vestibular nerve to prevent information about movement from getting to the brain. The vestibular nerve sends balance and movement information from your inner ear to the brain. This procedure usually improves vertigo and keeps hearing in the diseased ear.
- ***Endolymphatic duct blockage (EDB)*** is a relatively new treatment option for Ménière's (2024). In this surgery, the endolymphatic duct is identified and is then blocked with a titanium clip. It has promising results for a *complete treatment* of Ménière's disease. There are no significant complications or adverse effects and there is no hearing loss due to the surgery.

Alternative Treatments

Aside from making adjustments to the diet and lifestyle, there are few natural options available to manage Ménière's disease.

Some herbs, such as ginger root and ginkgo biloba may provide relief from vertigo symptoms in some people. However, according to the Medical research, no evidence supports using herbal supplements, acupuncture, or acupressure to treat Ménière's. Herbal supplements may also interact with existing medications. People who wish to try these remedies should check with a doctor before taking them.

Does Ménière's disease go away?

Ménière's disease *may* go away for months or years. You might hear people on social media groups say they are in remission. To me, this insinuates that it will never return, but it has a very high likelihood of returning. I like to call it dormant when you have relief from symptoms for a specified time. Generally, Ménière's disease vertigo happens in clusters, where you have an onslaught of vertigo and tinnitus and hearing loss and brain fog and nausea all within a number of weeks or months, before it clears for a little while. Doctors, specialists and researchers all agree that Ménière's disease is a chronic illness that most probably never really goes away.

Having said that, I do know of people officially diagnosed, with whose Ménière's symptoms have never returned.

There is always, always hope.

Do You Really Have Ménière's Disease?

In 2014, when I volunteered to be a Ménière's research subject at the University of Queensland's Brain and Mind Centre, the researcher told me a story about a woman who also volunteered to be a research subject. During the rigorous testing required for the research, it was discovered that she did not in fact have Ménière's disease, but BPPV, which is easily fixed, and the woman had put up with vertigo for twenty years! This is why I always ask, *do you really have Ménière's disease?* What if you have a condition that can be fixed? Make sure you have an ENT and MD testing to rule out other conditions like:

• *Benign Paroxysmal Positional Vertigo* (BPPV) – where certain head movements trigger vertigo - treatment - the Epley Manoeuvre

• *Migraines Associated Vertigo* (MAV) – severe headaches, these headaches can also not present with pain.

• *Labyrinthitis* – an inner ear infection

• *Vestibular Neuronitis* – inflammation of the vestibular nerve

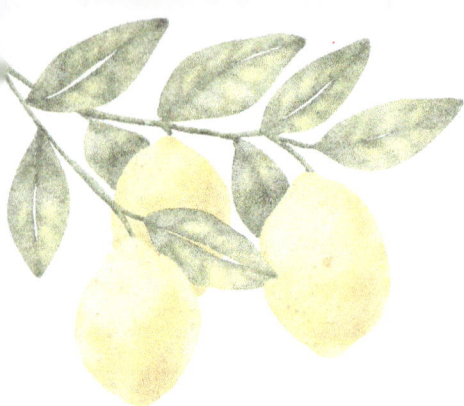

Dear Me,

Forgive others when they don't understand my life with Ménière's disease - the vertigo, the tinnitus, the hearing loss, the anxiety, the unpredictability of my social life, the depression, the grief, the PTSD.

Forgive myself as well.

Love, Me

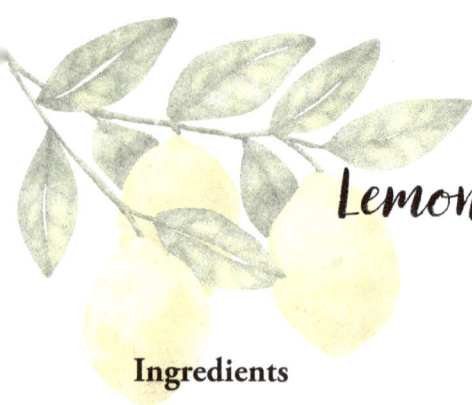

Lemon Cupcakes

Ingredients

150g unsalted butter
150g caster sugar
175g self-raising flour
3 eggs
1 tsp vanilla extract
1 lemon zested

Icing

150g unsalted butter softened
250g icing sugar
1 tsp vanilla extract
2 tsp hot water
1 lemon zested

Directions

1. Preheat the oven to 180C.
2. Line a 12-section bun tray with cupcake cases.
3. Place all of the ingredients into a bowl or food mixer, and beat until creamy and light.
4. Evenly divide the mixture into the 12 cake cases.
5. Bake for 18-20 minutes until they have risen and are firm to touch.
6. Cool on a wire rack.

Icing

1. Place the butter and icing sugar into a bowl or food mixer, and beat well until smooth and creamy.
2. Add the vanilla extract, the hot water and the grated lemon rind. Beat again until smooth.
3. Once the cupcakes have cooled, spoon or pipe the mixture evenly onto them.

Notes (thoughts, photos, tweaks to recipe)

Secret Women's Business

'**A** question for the women…' often pops up in Ménière's disease social media. Men instantly scroll past and pretend it doesn't exist. Some women do too.

My dear mum is eighty-two years old this year, and her generation is one to never talk about women's body parts or women's bodily functions. Or sex. Or child birth. Or urinary incontinence. Or weak pelvic floor muscles. Count yourself lucky if your mum is able to talk openly about being a woman.

I recently sat in on a Year 7 (12 and 13 year olds) Sex Education Class as a supervising teacher. At my age I thought I could not be shocked. Well … was I in for a surprise. Mostly because my sex education, in the late 1970s consisted of mum giving me the book to read by myself, "Where Did I Come From?" And I skipped all the rude pages. In the open discussions in the class, no body part was off limit. Whether you were biologically a male of female, everything was discussed in front of everyone, the presenter declaring 'Boys, you need to know this too!' when talking about changes in females, from how far the vagina can stretch with penile penetration, to giving birth, to monthly blood flow and painful periods and mood changes. The girls didn't miss out, learning about male reproductive parts, how they work and change. All the anatomically correct language was used for the body. There was no blushing or shame. The answers were all delivered in a factual and respectful way. That generation is winning.

Which brings me back to womanhood and the flourish of anecdotal stories of women asking whether their Ménière's symptoms worsen at points in their menstrual cycle, or during pregnancy, or during perimenopause or menopause.

Our state of being a woman adds an extra layer of complexity onto the already complex Ménière's disease, for sure.

Hormonal Research linking to Ménière's Disease

If you research hormonal effects on Ménière's disease on the Internet, there is little recent data on the topic. Little research, fullstop. In fact, you can garner more information from social media like *Facebook* and *Reddit* than in the medical journals. Real life anecdotes.

However, the few articles that do exist, acknowledge that hormonal changes in women can result in a change of fluid movement that can result in a Ménière's attack.

Ménière's and Menstruation

The menstrual cycle has four phases:

- Menstruation – commonly known as a period.
- The follicular phase - starts on the first day of your period and lasts for 13 to 14 days, ending in ovulation
- Ovulation - when a mature egg is released from an ovary and moves along a fallopian tube towards your uterus. This usually happens once each month, about two weeks before your next period. Ovulation can last from 16 to 32 hours.
- The luteal phase - the lining of the uterus thickening in preparation for pregnancy

According to Ménière's Organisation UK, 70% of menstruating women noted a worsening of the MD symptoms during the premenstrual period (one or two weeks before their period).

However, another study found a decrease in vertigo during the premenstrual period.

Typical of Ménière's to throw a curve ball into the research.

Of the women who had an exacerbation of symptoms, there was a measurable difference in the audiometric function, with hearing significantly worse during the premenstrual period.

Have you noticed that?

It is believed that during the premenstrual period, the fluid in the inner ear may be responsive to changes in hormones. When estrogen is low, as in the premenstrual phase of the menstrual cycle, there is more fluid accumulation in the inner ear, which goes with the fact that some women experience increased water and salt retention around the time of their period. This is due to an increase in the hormone progesterone. Progesterone activates the hormone aldosterone, which causes the kidneys to retain water and salt.

Makes sense. So we aren't imagining our changes in symptoms that accompany our cycles.

Your story

Changes in your Ménière's symptoms during your monthly cycle.

Possible Solutions

It is important to note that when investigating your exacerbation of your Ménière's symptoms with your monthly cycle, you will need to find out what treatments may help you, and **talk to your specialist or doctor about it**. Here are some suggestions from research that may help:

- take a diuretic in the premenstrual phase
- contraceptives (birth control) – oral or implanted
- increase betahistine beforehand if you have a predictable cycle, then drop back to usual maintenance afterward
- Period tracker – on paper or an app - monitoring symptoms across several menstrual cycles may help a person identify the specific cause, pattern or trigger
- hormone evaluation - you may benefit from a hormonal evaluation in the event that the hormonal imbalance contributes to your Ménière's symptoms.

The good news is that research studies have provided evidence that a unique relationship does exist between the menstrual cycle and Ménière's disease responses for some women. We are not just imagining things. I noted as I was reading research about Ménière's and menstruation that recommendations included "further research with larger samples and testing of different symptom management strategies for women of different perimenstrual symptom patterns". I'm yet to see any evidence of this further research. However, there was one study – "Effects of combined oral contraception containing drospirenone on premenstrual exacerbation of Ménière's disease: Preliminary study" that claimed to help with that time of the month. It was purely research though.

www.sciencedirect.com/science/article/abs/pii/S0301211518301106

Not everyone wants to take oral contraception though.

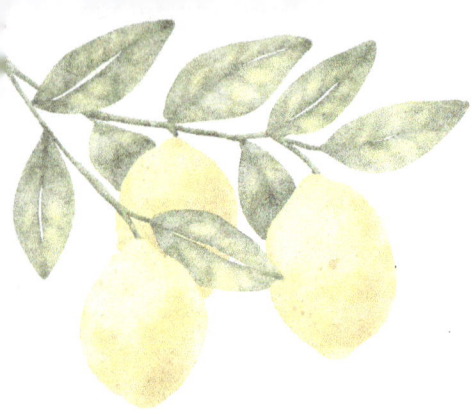

Monthly Period
and Symptom tracker

The next section of this book is a tracker for Ménière's symptoms each month. You may find patterns or triggers. Please add any other information to it that you need to, as we are all different. Be creative. Use colours, highlighters, or stick inspirations or whatever in the pages as well.

The tracker can also be used for perimenopause.

MONTH: January February March April May June July August September October November December

1	2	3	4
5	6	7	8
9	10	11	12
13	14	15	16
17	18	19	20
21	22	23	24
25	26	27	28
29	30	31	

Symptoms:

Tinnitus (T)	Vertigo (V)	Drop Attack (DA)	Nausea (N)
Anxiety (A)	Brain Fog (BF)	Hearing Loss (HL)	Hyperacusis (H)
Fatigue (F)	Balance (B)	Co-ordination (C)	Stress (S)
Headache (H)	Migraine (M)	Nystagmus (Ny)	Disequilibrium (D)
Ear Fullness/ Pressure/Pain (E)	Vision Difficulties (V)	Physical Impairment (P)	Vestibular Migraine (VM)
Vomiting (V)	Depression (Dep)	BPPV* (BPPV)	Diarrhea (Di)
PPPD* (PP)	Jaw Click/Pain (J)	Neck Pain (Np)	Motion Sensitivity (Ms)
Sweating (Sw)	Speech Difficulty (Sp)	Bloating (Bl)	Motion Sensitivity (Ms)
Cramping (Cr)	Breast Pain (Bp)	Moody (My)	Menstruation***

What part of the cycle did your symptoms start?
Premenstrual? (1 or 2 weeks prior) During menstruation? After?
Tinnitus: When? Pre? During? After? Loudness Scale: 1 2 3 4 5
Possible Menstruation & Ménière's Patterns. What I noticed.

Duration of Vertigo _____ minutes _____ hours_____ days
Severity of Vertigo 1   2   3   4   5 - I HATE you, vertigo!
New Symptoms? _____

What Helped Me?

Medication/s & Time Taken		Other	
		Prayer	Rest
		Meditation	Friend/s
		Self-care	Family
		Exercise	Pet/s
		Mindfulness	Vestibular Rehab
		Gratitude	Hearing Device

What I Accomplished this Month - Something to Celebrate! ♡

Three Things I am Thankful for This Month:

1.
2.
3.

MONTH: January February March April May June July August September October November December

1	2	3	4
5	6	7	8
9	10	11	12
13	14	15	16
17	18	19	20
21	22	23	24
25	26	27	28
29	30	31	

Symptoms:

Tinnitus (T)	Vertigo (V)	Drop Attack (DA)	Nausea (N)
Anxiety (A)	Brain Fog (BF)	Hearing Loss (HL)	Hyperacusis (H)
Fatigue (F)	Balance (B)	Co-ordination (C)	Stress (S)
Headache (H)	Migraine (M)	Nystagmus (Ny)	Disequilibrium (D)
Ear Fullness/Pressure/Pain (E)	Vision Difficulties (V)	Physical Impairment (P)	Vestibular Migraine (VM)
Vomiting (V)	Depression (Dep)	BPPV* (BPPV)	Diarrhea (Di)
PPPD* (PP)	Jaw Click/Pain (J)	Neck Pain (Np)	Motion Sensitivity (Ms)
Sweating (Sw)	Speech Difficulty (Sp)	Bloating (Bl)	
Cramping (Cr)	Breast Pain (Bp)	Moody (My)	Menstruation***

What part of the cycle did your symptoms start?
Premenstrual? (1 or 2 weeks prior) **During menstruation? After?**
Tinnitus: When? Pre? During? After? **Loudness Scale:** 1 2 3 4 5
Possible Menstruation & Ménière's Patterns. What I noticed.

_____
_____
_____
_____
_____
_____
_____

Duration of Vertigo _____ minutes _____ hours____ days
Severity of Vertigo 1 2 3 4 5 - I HATE you, vertigo!
New Symptoms? _____
_____

What Helped Me?

Medication/s & Time Taken		Other	
		Prayer	Rest
		Meditation	Friend/s
		Self-care	Family
		Exercise	Pet/s
		Mindfulness	Vestibular Rehab
		Gratitude	Hearing Device

What I Accomplished this Month - Something to Celebrate! ♡

_____
_____

Three Things I am Thankful for This Month:

1.
2.
3.

MONTH: January February March April May June July August September October November December

1	2	3	4
5	6	7	8
9	10	11	12
13	14	15	16
17	18	19	20
21	22	23	24
25	26	27	28
29	30	31	

Symptoms:

Tinnitus (T)	Vertigo (V)	Drop Attack (DA)	Nausea (N)
Anxiety (A)	Brain Fog (BF)	Hearing Loss (HL)	Hyperacusis (H)
Fatigue (F)	Balance (B)	Co-ordination (C)	Stress (S)
Headache (H)	Migraine (M)	Nystagmus (Ny)	Disequilibrium (D)
Ear Fullness/ Pressure/Pain (E)	Vision Difficulties (V)	Physical Impairment (P)	Vestibular Migraine (VM)
Vomiting (V)	Depression (Dep)	BPPV* (BPPV)	Diarrhea (Di)
PPPD* (PP)	Jaw Click/Pain (J)	Neck Pain (Np)	Motion Sensitivity (Ms)
Sweating (Sw)	Speech Difficulty (Sp)	Bloating (Bl)	
Cramping (Cr)	Breast Pain (Bp)	Moody (My)	Menstruation***

What part of the cycle did your symptoms start?
Premenstrual? (1 or 2 weeks prior) During menstruation? After?
Tinnitus: When? Pre? During? After? Loudness Scale: 1 2 3 4 5
Possible Menstruation & Ménière's Patterns. What I noticed.

_____
_____
_____
_____
_____
_____

Duration of Vertigo _____ minutes _____ hours____ days
Severity of Vertigo 1   2   3   4   5 - I HATE you, vertigo!
New Symptoms? _____

What Helped Me?

Medication/s & Time Taken		Other	
		Prayer	Rest
		Meditation	Friend/s
		Self-care	Family
		Exercise	Pet/s
		Mindfulness	Vestibular Rehab
		Gratitude	Hearing Device

What I Accomplished this Month - Something to Celebrate! ♡

_____
_____

Three Things I am Thankful for This Month:

1.
2.
3.

1	2	3	4
5	6	7	8
9	10	11	12
13	14	15	16
17	18	19	20
21	22	23	24
25	26	27	28
29	30	31	

Symptoms:

Tinnitus (T)	Vertigo (V)	Drop Attack (DA)	Nausea (N)
Anxiety (A)	Brain Fog (BF)	Hearing Loss (HL)	Hyperacusis (H)
Fatigue (F)	Balance (B)	Co-ordination (C)	Stress (S)
Headache (H)	Migraine (M)	Nystagmus (Ny)	Disequilibrium (D)
Ear Fullness/ Pressure/Pain (E)	Vision Difficulties (V)	Physical Impairment (P)	Vestibular Migraine (VM)
Vomiting (V)	Depression (Dep)	BPPV* (BPPV)	Diarrhea (Di)
PPPD* (PP)	Jaw Click/Pain (J)	Neck Pain (Np)	Motion Sensitivity (Ms)
Sweating (Sw)	Speech Difficulty (Sp)	Bloating (Bl)	
Cramping (Cr)	Breast Pain (Bp)	Moody (My)	Menstruation***

What part of the cycle did your symptoms start?
Premenstrual? (1 or 2 weeks prior) **During menstruation? After?**
Tinnitus: When? Pre? During? After? **Loudness Scale:** 1 2 3 4 5
Possible Menstruation & Ménière's Patterns. What I noticed.

_____
_____
_____
_____
_____
_____
_____

Duration of Vertigo _____ minutes _____ hours_____ days
Severity of Vertigo 1 2 3 4 5 - I HATE you, vertigo!
New Symptoms? _____

What Helped Me?

Medication/s & Time Taken		Other	
		Prayer	Rest
		Meditation	Friend/s
		Self-care	Family
		Exercise	Pet/s
		Mindfulness	Vestibular Rehab
		Gratitude	Hearing Device

What I Accomplished this Month - Something to Celebrate! ♡

_____

_____

Three Things I am Thankful for This Month:

1.
2.
3.

MONTH: January February March April May June July August September October November December

1	2	3	4
5	6	7	8
9	10	11	12
13	14	15	16
17	18	19	20
21	22	23	24
25	26	27	28
29	30	31	

Symptoms:

Tinnitus (T)	Vertigo (V)	Drop Attack (DA)	Nausea (N)
Anxiety (A)	Brain Fog (BF)	Hearing Loss (HL)	Hyperacusis (H)
Fatigue (F)	Balance (B)	Co-ordination (C)	Stress (S)
Headache (H)	Migraine (M)	Nystagmus (Ny)	Disequilibrium (D)
Ear Fullness/ Pressure/Pain (E)	Vision Difficulties (V)	Physical Impairment (P)	Vestibular Migraine (VM)
Vomiting (V)	Depression (Dep)	BPPV* (BPPV)	Diarrhea (Di)
PPPD* (PP)	Jaw Click/Pain (J)	Neck Pain (Np)	Motion Sensitivity (Ms)
Sweating (Sw)	Speech Difficulty (Sp)	Bloating (Bl)	
Cramping (Cr)	Breast Pain (Bp)	Moody (My)	Menstruation***

What part of the cycle did your symptoms start?
Premenstrual? (1 or 2 weeks prior) **During menstruation?   After?**
Tinnitus: When? Pre? During? After? **Loudness Scale:** 1 2 3 4 5
Possible Menstruation & Ménière's Patterns. What I noticed.

_____

_____

_____

_____

_____

_____

_____

Duration of Vertigo _____ minutes _____ hours____ days
Severity of Vertigo 1   2   3   4   5 - I HATE you, vertigo!
New Symptoms? _____

What Helped Me?

Medication/s & Time Taken		Other	
		Prayer	Rest
		Meditation	Friend/s
		Self-care	Family
		Exercise	Pet/s
		Mindfulness	Vestibular Rehab
		Gratitude	Hearing Device

What I Accomplished this Month - Something to Celebrate! ♀

_____

_____

_____

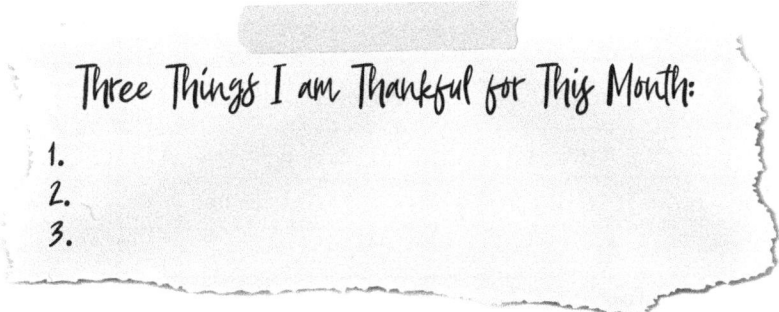

Three Things I am Thankful for This Month:

1.
2.
3.

1	2	3	4
5	6	7	8
9	10	11	12
13	14	15	16
17	18	19	20
21	22	23	24
25	26	27	28
29	30	31	

Symptoms:

Tinnitus (T)	Vertigo (V)	Drop Attack (DA)	Nausea (N)
Anxiety (A)	Brain Fog (BF)	Hearing Loss (HL)	Hyperacusis (H)
Fatigue (F)	Balance (B)	Co-ordination (C)	Stress (S)
Headache (H)	Migraine (M)	Nystagmus (Ny)	Disequilibrium (D)
Ear Fullness/ Pressure/Pain (E)	Vision Difficulties (V)	Physical Impairment (P)	Vestibular Migraine (VM)
Vomiting (V)	Depression (Dep)	BPPV* (BPPV)	Diarrhea (Di)
PPPD* (PP)	Jaw Click/Pain (J)	Neck Pain (Np)	Motion Sensitivity (Ms)
Sweating (Sw)	Speech Difficulty (Sp)	Bloating (Bl)	
Cramping (Cr)	Breast Pain (Bp)	Moody (My)	Menstruation***

What part of the cycle did your symptoms start?
Premenstrual? (1 or 2 weeks prior) **During menstruation?** **After?**
Tinnitus: When? Pre? During? After? **Loudness Scale:** 1 2 3 4 5
Possible Menstruation & Ménière's Patterns. What I noticed.

Duration of Vertigo _____ minutes _____ hours_____ days
Severity of Vertigo 1   2   3   4   5 - I HATE you, vertigo!
New Symptoms? _____

What Helped Me?

Medication/s & Time Taken		Other	
		Prayer	Rest
		Meditation	Friend/s
		Self-care	Family
		Exercise	Pet/s
		Mindfulness	Vestibular Rehab
		Gratitude	Hearing Device

What I Accomplished this Month - Something to Celebrate! ♡

Three Things I am Thankful for This Month:

1.
2.
3.

MONTH: January February March April May June July August September October November December

1	2	3	4
5	6	7	8
9	10	11	12
13	14	15	16
17	18	19	20
21	22	23	24
25	26	27	28
29	30	31	

Symptoms:

Tinnitus (T)	Vertigo (V)	Drop Attack (DA)	Nausea (N)
Anxiety (A)	Brain Fog (BF)	Hearing Loss (HL)	Hyperacusis (H)
Fatigue (F)	Balance (B)	Co-ordination (C)	Stress (S)
Headache (H)	Migraine (M)	Nystagmus (Ny)	Disequilibrium (D)
Ear Fullness/Pressure/Pain (E)	Vision Difficulties (V)	Physical Impairment (P)	Vestibular Migraine (VM)
Vomiting (V)	Depression (Dep)	BPPV* (BPPV)	Diarrhea (Di)
PPPD* (PP)	Jaw Click/Pain (J)	Neck Pain (Np)	Motion Sensitivity (Ms)
Sweating (Sw)	Speech Difficulty (Sp)	Bloating (Bl)	
Cramping (Cr)	Breast Pain (Bp)	Moody (My)	Menstruation***

What part of the cycle did your symptoms start?
Premenstrual? (1 or 2 weeks prior) During menstruation? After?
Tinnitus: When? Pre? During? After? Loudness Scale: 1 2 3 4 5
Possible Menstruation & Ménière's Patterns. What I noticed.

_____

_____

_____

_____

_____

_____

_____

Duration of Vertigo _____ minutes _____ hours_____ days
Severity of Vertigo 1   2   3   4   5 - I HATE you, vertigo!
New Symptoms? _____

_____

What Helped Me?

Medication/s & Time Taken		Other	
		Prayer	Rest
		Meditation	Friend/s
		Self-care	Family
		Exercise	Pet/s
		Mindfulness	Vestibular Rehab
		Gratitude	Hearing Device

What I Accomplished this Month - Something to Celebrate! ♡

_____

_____

_____

Three Things I am Thankful for This Month:

1.
2.
3.

MONTH: January February March April May June July August September October November December

1	2	3	4
5	6	7	8
9	10	11	12
13	14	15	16
17	18	19	20
21	22	23	24
25	26	27	28
29	30	31	

Symptoms:

Tinnitus (T)	Vertigo (V)	Drop Attack (DA)	Nausea (N)
Anxiety (A)	Brain Fog (BF)	Hearing Loss (HL)	Hyperacusis (H)
Fatigue (F)	Balance (B)	Co-ordination (C)	Stress (S)
Headache (H)	Migraine (M)	Nystagmus (Ny)	Disequilibrium (D)
Ear Fullness/ Pressure/Pain (E)	Vision Difficulties (V)	Physical Impairment (P)	Vestibular Migraine (VM)
Vomiting (V)	Depression (Dep)	BPPV* (BPPV)	Diarrhea (Di)
PPPD* (PP)	Jaw Click/Pain (J)	Neck Pain (Np)	Motion Sensitivity (Ms)
Sweating (Sw)	Speech Difficulty (Sp)	Bloating (Bl)	
Cramping (Cr)	Breast Pain (Bp)	Moody (My)	Menstruation***

What part of the cycle did your symptoms start?
Premenstrual? (1 or 2 weeks prior) **During menstruation?   After?**
Tinnitus: When? Pre? During? After? **Loudness Scale:** 1 2 3 4 5
Possible Menstruation & Ménière's Patterns. What I noticed.

Duration of Vertigo _____ minutes _____ hours_____ days
Severity of Vertigo 1   2   3   4   5 - I HATE you, vertigo!
New Symptoms? _____

What Helped Me?

Medication/s & Time Taken		Other	
		Prayer	Rest
		Meditation	Friend/s
		Self-care	Family
		Exercise	Pet/s
		Mindfulness	Vestibular Rehab
		Gratitude	Hearing Device

What I Accomplished this Month - Something to Celebrate! ♡

Three Things I am Thankful for This Month:

1.
2.
3.

MONTH: January February March April May June July August September October November December

1	2	3	4
5	6	7	8
9	10	11	12
13	14	15	16
17	18	19	20
21	22	23	24
25	26	27	28
29	30	31	

Symptoms:

Tinnitus (T)	Vertigo (V)	Drop Attack (DA)	Nausea (N)
Anxiety (A)	Brain Fog (BF)	Hearing Loss (HL)	Hyperacusis (H)
Fatigue (F)	Balance (B)	Co-ordination (C)	Stress (S)
Headache (H)	Migraine (M)	Nystagmus (Ny)	Disequilibrium (D)
Ear Fullness/ Pressure/Pain (E)	Vision Difficulties (V)	Physical Impairment (P)	Vestibular Migraine (VM)
Vomiting (V)	Depression (Dep)	BPPV* (BPPV)	Diarrhea (Di)
PPPD* (PP)	Jaw Click/Pain (J)	Neck Pain (Np)	Motion Sensitivity (Ms)
Sweating (Sw)	Speech Difficulty (Sp)	Bloating (Bl)	
Cramping (Cr)	Breast Pain (Bp)	Moody (My)	Menstruation***

What part of the cycle did your symptoms start?
Premenstrual? (1 or 2 weeks prior) During menstruation? After?
Tinnitus: When? Pre? During? After? Loudness Scale: 1 2 3 4 5
Possible Menstruation & Ménière's Patterns. What I noticed.

_____

_____

_____

_____

_____

_____

_____

Duration of Vertigo _____ minutes _____ hours_____ days
Severity of Vertigo 1 2 3 4 5 - I HATE you, vertigo!
New Symptoms? _____

What Helped Me?

Medication/s & Time Taken		Other	
		Prayer	Rest
		Meditation	Friend/s
		Self-care	Family
		Exercise	Pet/s
		Mindfulness	Vestibular Rehab
		Gratitude	Hearing Device

What I Accomplished this Month - Something to Celebrate! ♡

_____

_____

Three Things I am Thankful for This Month:

1.
2.
3.

MONTH: January February March April May June July August September October November December

1	2	3	4
5	6	7	8
9	10	11	12
13	14	15	16
17	18	19	20
21	22	23	24
25	26	27	28
29	30	31	

Symptoms:

Tinnitus (T)	Vertigo (V)	Drop Attack (DA)	Nausea (N)
Anxiety (A)	Brain Fog (BF)	Hearing Loss (HL)	Hyperacusis (H)
Fatigue (F)	Balance (B)	Co-ordination (C)	Stress (S)
Headache (H)	Migraine (M)	Nystagmus (Ny)	Disequilibrium (D)
Ear Fullness/ Pressure/Pain (E)	Vision Difficulties (V)	Physical Impairment (P)	Vestibular Migraine (VM)
Vomiting (V)	Depression (Dep)	BPPV* (BPPV)	Diarrhea (Di)
PPPD* (PP)	Jaw Click/Pain (J)	Neck Pain (Np)	Motion Sensitivity (Ms)
Sweating (Sw)	Speech Difficulty (Sp)	Bloating (Bl)	
Cramping (Cr)	Breast Pain (Bp)	Moody (My)	Menstruation***

What part of the cycle did your symptoms start?
Premenstrual? (1 or 2 weeks prior) **During menstruation? After?**
Tinnitus: When? Pre? During? After? **Loudness Scale:** 1 2 3 4 5
Possible Menstruation & Ménière's Patterns. What I noticed.

_____
_____
_____
_____
_____
_____
_____

Duration of Vertigo _____ minutes _____ hours _____ days
Severity of Vertigo 1   2   3   4   5 - I HATE you, vertigo!
New Symptoms? _____

What Helped Me?

Medication/s & Time Taken		Other	
		Prayer	Rest
		Meditation	Friend/s
		Self-care	Family
		Exercise	Pet/s
		Mindfulness	Vestibular Rehab
		Gratitude	Hearing Device

What I Accomplished this Month - Something to Celebrate! ♡

_____
_____

Three Things I am Thankful for This Month:

1.
2.
3.

MONTH: January February March April May June July August September October November December

1	2	3	4
5	6	7	8
9	10	11	12
13	14	15	16
17	18	19	20
21	22	23	24
25	26	27	28
29	30	31	

Symptoms:

Tinnitus (T)	Vertigo (V)	Drop Attack (DA)	Nausea (N)
Anxiety (A)	Brain Fog (BF)	Hearing Loss (HL)	Hyperacusis (H)
Fatigue (F)	Balance (B)	Co-ordination (C)	Stress (S)
Headache (H)	Migraine (M)	Nystagmus (Ny)	Disequilibrium (D)
Ear Fullness/ Pressure/Pain (E)	Vision Difficulties (V)	Physical Impairment (P)	Vestibular Migraine (VM)
Vomiting (V)	Depression (Dep)	BPPV* (BPPV)	Diarrhea (Di)
PPPD* (PP)	Jaw Click/Pain (J)	Neck Pain (Np)	Motion Sensitivity (Ms)
Sweating (Sw)	Speech Difficulty (Sp)	Bloating (Bl)	
Cramping (Cr)	Breast Pain (Bp)	Moody (My)	Menstruation***

What part of the cycle did your symptoms start?
Premenstrual? (1 or 2 weeks prior) During menstruation? After?
Tinnitus: When? Pre? During? After? Loudness Scale: 1 2 3 4 5
Possible Menstruation & Ménière's Patterns. What I noticed.

_____

_____

_____

_____

_____

_____

_____

Duration of Vertigo _____ minutes _____ hours _____ days
Severity of Vertigo 1 2 3 4 5 - I HATE you, vertigo!
New Symptoms? _____

What Helped Me?

Medication/s & Time Taken		Other	
		Prayer	Rest
		Meditation	Friend/s
		Self-care	Family
		Exercise	Pet/s
		Mindfulness	Vestibular Rehab
		Gratitude	Hearing Device

What I Accomplished the Month - Something to Celebrate! ♡

_____

_____

Three Things I am Thankful for This Month:

1.
2.
3.

MONTH: January February March April May June July August September October November December

1	2	3	4
5	6	7	8
9	10	11	12
13	14	15	16
17	18	19	20
21	22	23	24
25	26	27	28
29	30	31	

Symptoms:

Tinnitus (T)	Vertigo (V)	Drop Attack (DA)	Nausea (N)
Anxiety (A)	Brain Fog (BF)	Hearing Loss (HL)	Hyperacusis (H)
Fatigue (F)	Balance (B)	Co-ordination (C)	Stress (S)
Headache (H)	Migraine (M)	Nystagmus (Ny)	Disequilibrium (D)
Ear Fullness/ Pressure/Pain (E)	Vision Difficulties (V)	Physical Impairment (P)	Vestibular Migraine (VM)
Vomiting (V)	Depression (Dep)	BPPV* (BPPV)	Diarrhea (Di)
PPPD* (PP)	Jaw Click/Pain (J)	Neck Pain (Np)	Motion Sensitivity (Ms)
Sweating (Sw)	Speech Difficulty (Sp)	Bloating (Bl)	
Cramping (Cr)	Breast Pain (Bp)	Moody (My)	Menstruation***

What part of the cycle did your symptoms start?
Premenstrual? (1 or 2 weeks prior) During menstruation? After?
Tinnitus: When? Pre? During? After? Loudness Scale: 1 2 3 4 5
Possible Menstruation & Ménière's Patterns. What I noticed.

_____
_____
_____
_____
_____
_____
_____

Duration of Vertigo _____ minutes _____ hours_____ days
Severity of Vertigo 1 2 3 4 5 - I HATE you, vertigo!
New Symptoms? _____
_____

What Helped Me?

Medication/s & Time Taken		Other	
		Prayer	Rest
		Meditation	Friend/s
		Self-care	Family
		Exercise	Pet/s
		Mindfulness	Vestibular Rehab
		Gratitude	Hearing Device

What I Accomplished the Month - Something to Celebrate! ♡

_____
_____

Three Things I am Thankful for This Month:

1.
2.
3.

Your Monthly Cycle

Notes

Your Plan of Action

Notes

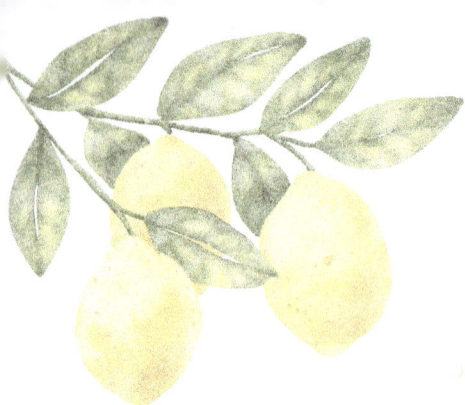

Dear Me,

My best is *different* everyday,
and that is okay.

Be *gentle* and *kind* to myself.

Love, Me

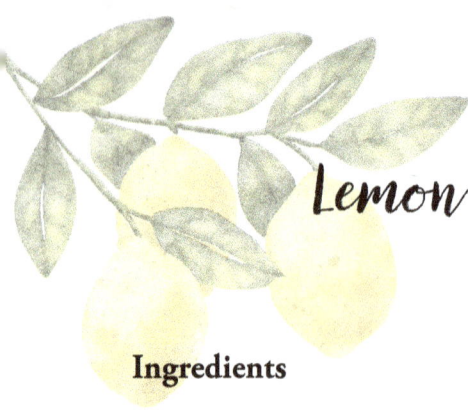

Lemon Cheesecake

Ingredients

750g cream cheese, at room temperature, chopped
315g (11/2 cups) caster sugar
3 tsp vanilla bean paste
5 eggs
410ml (1 2/3 cups) thickened cream
100g (2/3 cup) plain flour
75g (1/4 cup) bought lemon curd, plus extra, to serve
Whipped cream, to serve
Lemon halves, thinly sliced, to serve (optional)
Thinly sliced lemon rind, to serve (optional

Directions

1. Preheat oven to 180C/160C for fan forced.
Grease a 22cm spring-form pan.
Line the base and side with baking paper.
Place in a baking dish.

2. Use electric beaters to beat the cream cheese, sugar and
vanilla in a large bowl until smooth.
Add the eggs, 1 at a time, beating well after each addition.
Add the cream and flour.
Beat until smooth.

3. Pour the cream cheese mixture into the prepared pan.
Top with the lemon curd and use the back of a spoon to swirl

the curd through the cream cheese mixture to create a marbled effect. Pour enough boiling water into the baking dish to come halfway up the side of the pan.

Bake for 1 hour or until just set in the middle.

Turn off the oven. Remove the cheesecake from the baking dish. Return cheesecake to the oven with the door slightly ajar until cooled completely.

4. Place the cheesecake in the fridge for 2 hours or overnight to chill.

5. Top the cheesecake with whipped cream, extra lemon curd, and lemon slices and rind, if using, to serve.

Notes (thoughts, photos, tweaks to recipe)

Ménière's and Pregnancy

"Your dream came true, your very own little one,
your brand new life as a mother is about to begin.
The moment you breathe in that new baby smell,
you'll feel a love so fierce, it's like nothing
you've ever felt before."

B ecoming a mum can be exciting and overwhelming and everything in between. Sometimes your emotions are like all four seasons in one day. Being a mum is a significant life change that will be challenging at times, but also most beautifully rewarding.

Should I have a baby when I've got Ménière's disease?

Such a common question. And an important one.

And I might add how spoiled we are with connecting online with other women with Ménière's. We can ask any question, any time, and there will be someone who has gone through the journey before us who can pass on wisdom and advice. We are also spoiled by the increased knowledge that doctors have with medications and their effects on the unborn children.

Never, have I read anywhere online in Ménière's groups, where someone with Ménière's has regretted choosing to have a baby. That doesn't mean that the going is not tough. The going is tough for many mothers, Ménière's or not. It's just that having Ménière's as well means we have to prepare ahead for scenarios of vertigo that may come our way. You may breeze through pregnancy, birth and raising your beautiful children, or you may be more challenged.

It is interesting to note, that pregnancy can trigger Ménière's disease for the first time in a woman who has never had it before.

74

If the thought of being pregnant when you have Ménière's is daunting, or makes you a little scared, that's completely normal. But the good news is, you can be prepared, even if the baby wasn't planned.

Motherhood is amazing and so incredibly brave.

Research

While researching Ménière's and pregnancy online, I discovered that there's not a lot of information, or research studies done on the subject. I wasn't surprised.

But what they do know with 100% accuracy, is that Ménière's disease itself won't harm your baby, but it may cause extra stress, depending on the severity of your Ménière's symptoms.

And ... it may not.

Planning a pregnancy?

- Always seek advice from your doctor about medications
- Research
- Chat with other mums with Ménière's disease
- Weigh up the pros and cons for you and your partner
- Communicate with your healthcare provider, as well as your family, to plan ahead for attacks, and monitor your diet and overall health and stress level to stay as healthy as possible during pregnancy.

Already pregnant - unplanned?

Congratulations! And don't worry yourself unnecessarily about taking Ménière's medications without knowing about your baby. You're not the first this has happened to, and you won't be the last.

Many healthy babies have come into the world, regardless. Head to your doctor as soon as possible though, so you can discuss your pregnancy and what medications are safe.

When you feel that first little kick, and hear a heartbeat for the first time, you suddenly understand what it means to love someone more than your own life.

Medical Research on Ménière's and Pregnancy

"During pregnancy, the course of the Ménière's disease is poorly documented in the medical literature. Ménière's disease has been shown to be exacerbated in late luteal phase of the menstrual cycle, and hence, it may have some relation with hormonal changes which leads to fluid retention in the inner ear.[7] Ménière's disease or endolymphatic hydrops is a disorder of the inner ear where endolymphatic system is distended by endolymph. It is characterized by vertigo, sensorineural hearing loss, and aural fullness. In acute attack of Ménière's disease, dimenhydrinate and meclizine can be safely given to the pregnant women. Histamines and diuretics are usually avoided in pregnancy for treating Ménière's disease as it cause hypotension, hypovolemia, and decrease the cardiac output. In case of intractable vomiting, metaclopromide can be used.[8]"

https://journals.lww.com/mjdy/fulltext/2021/14040/otorhinolaryngological_manifestations_in_pregnant.3.aspx

"To date, few data have revealed that vertigo is exacerbated in patients with a previous history of Ménière's disease during pregnancy and some others have reported their onset to be associated with vestibular neuritis; however, there is a lack of information regarding this symptom throughout pregnancy [2]"

Pérez Rodríguez AF, Roche M, Larrañaga C: [Medical disorders and pregnancy. Gastrointestinal, neurological, cardiovascular and dermatological disorders]. An Sist Sanit Navar. 2009, 32 Suppl 1:135-57. 10.23938/ASSN.0186

"There are conflicting reports from pregnant women with Ménière's, some say their symptoms were at their worst during pregnancy, others say they had no symptoms at all. Conversely, some women with Ménière's report an improvement of their symptoms during pregnancy. This may be down to a prostaglandin called PGI2, which is increased during pregnancy, and has been shown to cause significant long term reduction in vertigo, completely controlling it."

https://www.menieres.org.uk/files/pdfs/Monaghan.pdf

The following excerpts are from Pregistry.com, by *Dr. Diego Wyszynski*, a leading pioneer in the field of maternal and neonatal health. He founded Pregistry with the vision of a world where all people and their health care providers have access to high-quality data about the reproductive risks of medicines and vaccines. You can read the full article at:

https://pregistry.com/report?action=pdf&rname=meniere-disease

How common is Ménière's disease during pregnancy?

... Often, the symptoms (of Ménière's disease) appear when a woman becomes pregnant for the first time. Women tend to develop Ménière's disease a little bit more frequently than men, and so its not unusual for the condition to co-exist with pregnancy.

Does Ménière's disease cause problems during pregnancy?

Many women have trouble with balance during the third trimester, as the belly grows very large and changes the body's centre of gravity. By interfering with the balance organs in the inner ears, Ménière's disease can exacerbate the problem adding to the risk of falling. The vertigo of Ménière's disease furthermore generates nausea, which can exacerbate pregnancy-induced nausea that is particularly troubling during the first trimester.

Does Ménière's disease during pregnancy cause problems for the baby?

No. The disease process underlying Ménière's disease is limited to the inner ear of the mother.

Having an infant son alerts me to the fact that every man, at one point, has peed on his own face
- Olivia Wilde

What to consider about taking medications when you are pregnant:

- Any risks to yourself and your baby if you do not treat the Ménière's disease
- The risks and benefits of each medication you use when you are pregnant
- The risks and benefits of each medication you use when you are breastfeeding

What should I know about using medication to treat Ménière's disease during pregnancy?

Medications for Ménière's disease fall into two categories: products used to stop or reduce attacks of vertigo, such as meclizine and promethazine, and agents that lower blood pressure, such as diuretics (eg, hydrochlorothiazide, acetazolamide) which are given to drive fluid out of the body in order to reduce the amount of fluid in the labyrinths. Other types of blood pressure-lowering drugs also are used, plus very severe cases of vertigo that do not improve with medication given by mouth can be treated by injection into the middle ear with an antibiotic called gentamicin. Sometimes, a group of anti-anxiety drugs called benzodiazepines is given as well to those who are anxious about a potential vertigo attack.

Who should NOT stop taking medication for Ménière's disease during pregnancy?

Anybody can try coping with the condition without medication. If you are already taking medication to control symptoms of Ménière's disease, in cooperation with your doctor you can try backing off from the drug, but since there are low risk medication options, ending drug treatment is generally not necessary.

What should I know about choosing a medication for my Ménière's disease during pregnancy?

The diuretic hydrochlorothiazide is thought to be relatively safe, but there is concern that acetazolamide may be harmful to the fetus, although studies have been limited. Studies suggest that these drugs are relatively safe during pregnancy when used correctly. Meclizine and promethazine are actually given commonly to treat nausea of pregnancy, as they are thought to be safe, so these are reasonable options for treating vertigo attacks as well. Benzodiazepines are best avoided as they may cause certain birth defects, if given during the first trimester.

Will I Pass Ménière's Disease on to My Children?

This is a very real concern for people with Ménière's, mothers and fathers alike. There can be a familial cause of Ménière's disease, but you will know that because there will be numerous relatives who also have the disease. Research from the Internet states that "most cases of Ménière disease are sporadic, which means they occur in people with no history of the disorder in their family. A small percentage of all cases have been reported to run in families. When the disorder is familial, it most often has an autosomal dominant pattern of inheritance".

https://medlineplus.gov/genetics/condition/meniere-disease/#inheritance

The good news is, researchers are making discoveries in leap and bounds with hereditary Ménière's. This quote is from research posted in May 2023, "As we have seen, the past couple of years has seen significant new developments in deciphering the root causes of Ménière's disease. As well as identifying those genes commonly associated with MD, an epigenetic component has also been elucidated. The genes shown to be involved suggest the likely involvement of proteins within the otolithic and tectorial membranes, as well as their links to stereocilia. Focal detachment of these membranes triggers spontaneous motility of hair cell bundles and random depolarization of hair cells, which may explain sudden onset of loud tinnitus or bouts of vertigo. The autoimmune aspects of the disease have also been further investigated, with the maintenance of a proinflammatory milieu in the inner ear a likely contributing factor in some patients. These developments provide us with several promising leads as potential therapeutic targets to help treat and, hopefully, eventually cure this debilitating and disabling suite of conditions". (bold added is mine)

World leading Ménière's disease researcher Professor Jose Antonio Lopez Escamez.

https://www.ncbi.nlm.nih.gov/pmc/articles/PMC10241347/

Now That You're Pregnant

The moment a child is born, the mother is also born. She never existed before. The woman existed, but the mother never. A mother is something absolutely new -
Bhagwan Shree Rajneesh

Congratulations! I am beyond excited for you, and a little jealous I have to add. When I was pregnant (3x) I didn't know any women with Ménière's, and there was no literature about Ménière's, let alone Ménière's and pregnancy! I had no Internet access back in 1995, and definitely no social media.

My story

Baby #1- It's a boy!

I was twenty-nine when my husband and I became serious about having a baby. The only Ménière's symptom I had was a full ear feeling, like I had water stuck in the canal of my ear, although there was no water in it. I hadn't experienced the vertigo of Ménière's, and I hadn't been diagnosed with it, yet. My ENT doctor was waiting to see what symptoms I would get next.

I didn't know anyone else with Ménière's disease in the 1990s, except my 60-year-old father-in-law. I never saw him ill, even though I had known him for eleven years by then. It was like there was nothing wrong with him. He had hearing aids and could hear very well. When my ENT suggested Ménière's, I did not know how severe and life changing it could be. I had no access to information about Ménière's. We had no Internet. The only medical research I could do was by going to a library, or by buying medical books - which I didn't do. Why would I when my father-in-law handled it so well?

Pregnancy number one was a breeze for me, except for nausea in the first three months. My left blocked ear cleared like it never had anything wrong with it! What Ménière's disease?

The birth went well, and post postpartum was as expected.

But when bubs was four months old, I was hit with my first vertigo attack. Two hours long. Violent and unrelenting. I still remember it to this day how shocked I was by its ferocity. Thankfully it hit on Saturday, when my husband was home.

My doctor gave me Stemetil to take for nausea.

I had no more vertigo attacks after that, and my ear felt good. I returned to teaching when bubs was nine months old, and still no vertigo attacks.

Ménière's symptoms before pregnancy:
• blocked/full ear

Ménière's symptoms during pregnancy:
- none

Ménière's symptoms postpartum: (6-8 weeks after birth):
- none
- when bubs was four months old I did have my very first vertigo attack

"I don't want to sleep like a baby, I want to sleep like my husband." — Unknown

Baby #2 - It's a girl!

Pregnancy number two was a also breeze for me, except for the morning sickness. I was still teaching full time and finished teaching four weeks before the due date.

Ménière's symptoms before pregnancy:
- fluctuating hearing occasionally. It didn't worry me though, as my hearing always returned to normal

Ménière's symptoms during pregnancy:
- none

Ménière's symptoms postpartum:
- none
- when bubs was about three months old, I started to have more vertigo attacks, but they were spaced out and did not worry me. My husband or my mum would come to help me out

Baby #3 - It's a boy!

Pregnancy number three was a breeze for me, except for the morning sickness, which was the worst of all my pregnancies. I went to my doctor for something to ease the nausea, and she gave me a script for Metoclopramide (Maxolon, Pramin). This medication has been used for a long time in pregnancy and has a long record of safety. It can be given as a tablet or an intravenous or intramuscular injection. It worked so well for the nausea that it made me feel like I wasn't pregnant anymore (terrifying) and so I stopped taking it, preferring the nausea knowing it was my body's normal response to being pregnant. Ménière's wasn't first and foremost in my mind, as I hadn't really had many vertigo attacks, and I also had the distraction of a three year old and one year old to care for.

Ménière's symptoms before pregnancy:
- a little fluctuating hearing
- two vertigo attacks some time after baby number two was born
- some fluctuating tinnitus

Ménière's symptoms during pregnancy:
- tinnitus
- two minor vertigo attacks. No medication was taken for the vertigo due to being off all medications

Ménière's symptoms postpartum:
- two days after the birth I had vertigo in hospital. It was a very gentle spin, nevertheless it was still vertigo. I was given an injection of Stemetil as bubs was being fed baby formula

Then two weeks later, with a three year old, a one year old and a two week old baby, I was hit with a bad vertigo attack. I managed to stagger to the wall phone as best as I could, and called my mum, who dropped everything she was doing and raced over to my house to take over everything while I lay on the bed staring at one flower on the wall and trying not to vomit.

When she couldn't settle my crying newborn, she laid him down behind me and all I could do was not move my head, and reach behind me to touch him and talk to him (while trying not to vomit) to try and soothe him. It was heartbreaking, and is something I will never forget, and eternally thankful to my mum for doing her best to help me and my babies.

In my third baby's first year, I did have more vertigo attacks. I believe the vertigo was exacerbated by:

- having three babies with reflux, and were difficult to feed
- the stress of having a three year old, one year old and new baby
- the lack of sleep, as you would expect

I also believe I was going through the grief process with the diagnosis of Ménière's, and that the full impact of having the disease was making itself felt.

When a heavy sadness wouldn't leave me, and my anxiety was sky high, I finally went to my doctor to ask for help.

She looked at me and my tears, and said, 'I'm not surprised you feel this way after everything you have been through!' She was referring to my Ménière's, the birth of my daughter, who had stopped moving in utero, and it was a real possibility that she would be still born, and when she was born by c-section, she had seizures afterward due to lack or oxygen and swelling of the brain.

My beautiful girl couldn't be given a positive outlook, and she was a difficult crying baby. Difficult to feed. A projectile vomiter. A terrible sleeper. Yet, in all of her baby photos, she is smiling.

So many prayers at her birth were said, the moment she was born, and the weeks afterward.

She was meant to have cerebral palsy, not walk, and have a very short attention span.

Well, she proved the doctors wrong. She has a very long attention span, was a rep touch football player, is an incredible artist, has a double degree from university and now teaches secondary students.

We also discovered when she had surgery at 3 years of age, that she wasn't getting enough oxygen while sleeping (she was a terrible snorer!). Once she had her tonsils and adenoids out, she slept beautifully, and like my dad said, 'The nice Claire is here now!' Here crankiness had been caused by breathing difficulties while she slept, meaning she was feeling tired all the time!

You know, when my doctor said, I'm not surprised you feel this way after everything you've been through, it was like a weight was lifted off my shoulders instantly. Just those confirming words meant the world to me. I am so thankful to have an empathetic, caring doctor like her.

She gave me a script for Cipramil. It was an anti-anxiety and anti-depressant, and when the medication kicked in, life was suddenly so much easier to deal with. It was like a hand reaching down to help me up, so I could get on with life again. I could change my mindset and my days were filled with more light a wonderful moments.

I guess your take-away from my baby story is don't wait to ask for help. You don't have to suffer. You don't have to dwell in that place of deep sadness. If you do need an anti-depressant, you don't have to go telling people. It's your business. It can be a life changer for you. It was for me.

> *"It's OK to be grumpy sometimes, to have bad days to struggle, to make mistakes, to say the wrong thing, feel overwhelmed and under-appreciated, to be out-of-sorts and sort-of-over-it all. It's ok for us big humans, and it's ok for our little humans, too. After all, we're all humans, right? How else will our little humans learn that it's okay to be human? Remember, we're imperfect humans growing imperfect humans in an imperfect world, and that's perfectly okay." – L.R. Knost*

Returning to You

You're pregnant. You've had it confirmed by your doctor, and you've made an action plan to monitor your diet and overall health and stress level to stay as healthy as possible during pregnancy, and after the birth.

During Pregnancy

There is no one-size-fits-all to managing Ménière's disease during pregnancy as the symptoms of Ménière's can differ from one person to another.

There are, however, some general suggestions that might help:

- *Avoiding trigger foods and drinks, such as caffeine, and salt.* If you suspect that particular food or drink is triggering your symptoms, it may be worth avoiding it during pregnancy. You will be familiar with this type of food trigger patterning from having Ménière's before you were pregnant.
- *Exercise.* Please consult your doctor before starting any new exercises, in case they are not suitable for pregnancy. Exercise has been proven to help to reduce stress and improve balance. Walking is always my go to for exercise, as I can enjoy the quiet time and breathing in of nature. Even just a stroll around my neighbourhood. I find it calming and grounding. Like resetting.
- *Sleeping position.* Experts recommend sleeping on the left side during pregnancy from 28 weeks until birth, to increase blood flow to the uterus and Fetus. Back sleeping can cause back pain and increase pressure on the heart. Lying on your back also puts pressure on major blood vessels, and can reduce the flow of blood to your uterus, and restricts your baby's oxygen supply. This can affect their heart rate. Consider using pillows for support. They can make adjusting your sleep position during pregnancy easier and help you get better sleep.

https://www.sleepfoundation.org/pregnancy/pregnancy-sleep-positions
https://www.pregnancybirthbaby.org.au/sleep-during-pregnancy

You will need more sleep than usual when you're pregnant. Your body is terribly busy creating a brand new human being. It's got the most important job in the world to do. But, hey, if your sleep isn't refreshing, or you're awake during the night more often, or if you work, or have other children and responsibilities, perhaps these suggestions may help to sneak in some extra ZZZZZZs:

- ❧ Take a nap during the daytime
- ❧ Have a rest as much as you can during the day
- ❧ Go for a walk in the late afternoon or early evening
- ❧ Relax before bed. Read. Have a bath. Listen to relaxing music. Watch some TV. Or do what you know will help you relax before bed
- ❧ Oh and ... go to bed earlier than usual

Yeah, nah did I hear you say? Those suggestions are impossible to do. I hear you perfectly! But maybe you can find a way to steal a few more ZZZZZs from time to time. Good luck!

- • *Manage stress*. While it may not be possible to completely eliminate stress, you might try relaxation techniques that work for you.

Ménière's Survival Packs

The thing about having Ménière's disease, is that you are always looking ahead to plan in case you have a vertigo attack, anywhere, anytime. That makes us super-planners! It's one of our superpowers.

Before you were pregnant, you probably took a survival kit with you everywhere, just in case of the worst case scenario of having an attack of vertigo in public. You probably had this:

My Normal Ménière's Survival Pack (when NOT pregnant)

- Stemetil, or other anti-nausea medication like Ondansetron
- Vomit bag/s
- Water
- Ear plugs
- Face wipes (for wiping vomit from around your mouth etc)
- Crackers, ginger
- A sweet in case of low blood sugar (jelly beans etc)
- Sunglasses for sun or light sensitivity
- List of phone numbers for either you to call for help, a friend, or a passerby
- An information card explaining Ménière's disease symptoms, or perhaps wear a medic-alert bracelet
- Change of clothes in the car

Ménière's Pregnancy Survival Pack

Your Ménière's Survival Pack will look a little different now that you are pregnant. People will probably try to tell you that your vertigo is just from being pregnant. But you will absolutely know the difference between pregnancy dizziness and Ménière's vertigo. You are the best just of what is happening with your body! In your survival pack in case of vertigo out in public:

- **Approved anti-nausea medication that is safe to take** while pregnant, *if* you choose to take some. Some women choose not to take any medication at all, unless it is life threatening.
- Vomit bag/s
- Water
- Ear plugs
- Face wipes (for wiping vomit from around your mouth etc)
- Crackers, ginger
- A sweet in case of low blood sugar (jelly beans etc)

- Sunglasses for sun or light sensitivity
- List of phone numbers for either you to call for help, a friend, or a passerby to help you
- An information card explaining Ménière's disease symptoms, or perhaps wear a medic-alert bracelet
- Change of clothes in the car

Before you go out, research where you are going:

- Will you feel safe? If not, will the stress impact your Ménière's symptoms?
- Are there toilets nearby?
- Is there an area where you can rest?
- Is there someone who will look out for you?

Don't let Ménière's shatter your dreams of becoming a mum. Pregnancy is only a short duration compared to the long life of your beautiful child/ren and the love and joy that they bring.

Ménière's and Feeding Your Baby

Welcome to the world, little one. Newborns don't need too much other than love, milk and warmth. When you have Ménière's disease you need to take into consideration whether you will need to take medication to keep vertigo under control. This may also define whether you breastfeed or formula feed.

There is a push for "breast is best", but you know what, breast isn't always best depending on your medical conditions or traumatic experiences. Some babies are difficult to breastfeed for a myriad of reasons. Mums deserve an informed choice about whether to breastfeed of formula feed. It all boils down to what is best for mum and the baby.

Nothing strikes fear in a new parent's heart like these words: Baby. Shark.

Breastfeeding

Breastmilk is the natural food for your baby.

"Human breastmilk is a living substance, so complex that scientists are still trying to find everything that is in it. Breastmilk varies from the beginning of the feed to the end of the feed, from day 1 to day 7 to day 30 and beyond. In short, your breastmilk is always exactly right for your baby!"

https://www.breastfeeding.asn.au/resources/whats-so-great-about-breastmilk

As you have read, breastmilk contains all the nutrients and factors your baby needs for their health and development.

Common Ménière's Medication and Breastmilk

The top concern for mums with Ménière's is what medications can they safely take while breastfeeding.

I have gathered the following information about medications and lactating from medical journals and studies.

***Please note: your first port of call about medication and breastfeeding is your doctor**, who has the latest information about your medications. The following information is to open discussions with your doctor. The best person to help your decided on what medication to take while breastfeeding, is your doctor.

Betahistine (Serc)

Serc® betahistine dihydrochloride
Consumer Medicine Information

Betahistine dihydrochloride is a commonly prescribed medication for Ménière's disease. It is an effective treatment for some Ménière's patients, but not all.

"Serc tablets contain the active ingredient betahistine dihydrochloride. Serc works by improving the blood flow of the inner ear and restoring it to normal. It also acts on the nerve endings in the inner ear to normalise the way in which the nerves respond to outside influences"

Tell your doctor if you are pregnant, intend to become pregnant. or are breastfeeding Your doctor can discuss the risks and benefits involved.

https://www.nhs.uk/medicines/betahistine/pregnancy-breastfeeding-and-fertility-while-taking-betahistine/

Effects on Breastfed Infants

There is not any information about taking betahistine while breastfeeding, but it's *likely it will get into breast milk. It is therefore recommended that you do not take this medicine while breastfeeding if possible.* *****Talk to your doctor or pharmacist who can advise you on how to manage your symptoms, and if other medicines might be better.**

If you do need to take betahistine while breastfeeding and you notice your baby is being sick or has diarrhoea, has a rash, seems lethargic, or is not feeding as well as usual, or you have any other concerns about your baby, contact your doctor, pharmacist, health visitor or midwife.

Prochlorperazine (Stemetil/ Buccastem)

Stemetil is a widely prescribed medication for people with Ménière's, taken while in active vertigo.

It's also a vestibular suppressant, stopping the incorrect messages coming from the inner ears to the eyes, to the spinal column and to the brain. When you take stemetil, the ears are no longer talking to the eyes, spinal column and brain as effectively.

Stemetil®
Prochlorperazine
Consumer Medicine Information

Stemetil belongs to a group of medicines called phenothiazines. It helps to correct chemical imbalances in the brain, allowing it to function correctly. These chemicals may also affect the parts of the brain which control nausea (feeling sick) and vomiting. Stemetil is used to treat nausea, vomiting and dizziness due to various causes, including migraine (severe headache).

Use of Stemetil is not recommended during breastfeeding. If you are breastfeeding or planning to breastfeed, talk to your doctor about using Stemetil.

It is recommended that you **do not breastfeed while taking Stemetil**, as it is not known whether Stemetil passes into breast milk.

Effects on Breastfed Infants

Based on minimal excretion of other phenothiazine derivatives, it appears that occasional *short-term use* of prochlorperazine for the treatment of nausea and vomiting poses little risk to the breastfed infant.

https://www.sps.nhs.uk/articles/safety-in-lactation-drugs-used-in-nausea-and-vertigo-2/

Domperidone and metoclopramide are considered to be compatible with breastfeeding as anti-emetics for short-term, low-dose use. Domperidone is considered to be the agent of choice for inadequate lactation because of its superior side effect profile, efficacy, and minimal passage into breast milk. Both should only be used short-term.

https://www.mayoclinic.org/drugs-supplements/meclizine-oral-route/precautions/drg-20075849?p=1

Meclizine Studies in women suggest that this medication poses minimal risk to the infant when used during breastfeeding.

Diuretics

Diuretics is often a first port of call for medications in trying to control vertigo attacks. According to the Mount Sinai Center for Hearing and Balance,

"Diuretics are the most commonly prescribed maintenance medications for Ménière's disease. Diuretics work by restricting the overproduction of fluid in the inner ear. Diuretics are long-term medications. They help reduce the number of vertigo attacks, and in some cases, they help stabilize hearing. Commonly used diuretics are Diamox (acetazolamide) and Dyazide (triamterene/HCTZ)."

https://www.ncbi.nlm.nih.gov/books/NBK500965/

Summary of Use during Lactation

Hydrochlorothiazide doses of 50 mg daily or less are *acceptable during lactation*. Intense diuresis with large doses may decrease breastmilk production.

Prednisone (Oral)

Prednisone is a common medication prescribed for Ménière's disease, to either prevent or stop vertigo, or to restore lost hearing. It works by decreasing inflammation, slowing down an overactive immune system, or replacing cortisol normally made in the body, which plays an important role in how the body responds to stress, illness, and injury. It belongs to a group of medications called steroids.

National Library of Medicine
Drugs and Lactation Database (LactMed®) Sept 2023
https://www.ncbi.nlm.nih.gov/books/NBK501077/

"Amounts of prednisone in breastmilk are very low. *No adverse effect have been reported in breastfed infants with maternal use of any corticosteroid during breastfeeding.* Although it is often recommended to avoid breastfeeding for 4 hours after a dose this maneuver is not necessary because prednisone milk levels are very low. High doses might occasionally cause temporary loss of milk supply."

Effects on breastfed Infants

None reported with prednisone or any other corticosteroid. In a prospective follow-up study, six nursing mothers reported taking prednisone (dosage unspecified) with no adverse infant effects.[5]

There are several reports of mothers breastfeeding during long-term use of corticosteroids with no adverse infant effects.

The National Transplantation Pregnancy Registry reports that as of December 2013, 124 women with transplants have taken prednisone while breastfeeding 169 infants for periods as long as 48 months, with no apparent infant harm.

A new baby smile is the most beautiful thing in the world, until you realize it came along with a smell.

Feeding Your Baby While Having Vertigo

The thought of having a disabling vertigo and having to feed your baby is a major stress for Ménière's mums. We love our babies and we want to make sure they are well-cared for.

First of all, and you will probably already know this and are well acquainted with the rule of elimination to find the cause of your vertigo. Let's look for simple solutions.

- Are you drinking enough water? Making breastmilk uses extra fluid, so you'll be more thirsty than usual. If you're not drinking enough fluids, dizziness is an effect of dehydration.
- Are you eating enough to keep your blood sugar steady throughout the day?
- Are you getting enough sleep?
- Is there any stress you can minimise?
- Have you got your other usual Ménière's symptoms that signify that your vertigo is caused my Ménière's?

Once you are certain it is the vertigo of the Ménière's Monster, what can you do?

Any of the following strategies can be tried, in any order. There may be other strategies you read about from other mums with Ménière's disease.

Breastfeeding Position

There's no right or wrong way to hold and feed your baby, and if vertigo hits before or while breastfeeding, you will need to find a position to feed in that is best for your vertigo. What's important is that you find the best position for your vertigo to be bearable. There are many breastfeeding websites that explain the different breastfeeding positions and you can consult a lactation specialist and/or ask other mums in Ménière's groups or breastfeeding groups.

Expressing Milk

Can you express your breastmilk and store it so bubs can be bottle-fed while you are having a vertigo attack by you or your partner and trusted person?

https://raisingchildren.net.au/babies/breastfeeding-bottle-feeding-solids/expressing-working-travelling/expressing-breastmilk

Freshly expressed breastmilk can be stored:

- at room temperature (26ºC or lower) for 6-8 hours
- in the fridge (5ºC or lower) for up to 72 hours – the best spot is the back of the fridge where it's coldest
- in the freezer compartment (-15ºC or lower) inside a fridge for 2 weeks
- in the freezer section (-18ºC or lower) of a fridge with a separate door for 3 months
- in a chest or upright deep freezer (-20ºC or lower) for 6-12 months.

Warm your container of breastmilk by placing it in warm water Don't use a microwave oven to thaw or warm the milk, because this destroys some of the components of breastmilk. It can also result in hot spots, which can burn a baby.

Pacifier

A pacifier can turn an angry, screaming baby into a calm baby, and can be a tool for you if you have vertigo while breastfeeding, to give you and your baby some space in a difficult situation. Once you feel able to breastfeed again, or your vertigo has settled somewhat, go back to breastfeeding.

Taking Medication

If your vertigo is debilitating, you can take some medications while breastfeeding, which I explored earlier in this chapter.

***But ensure you have discussed your medications with your doctor to be absolutely sure that what you would like to take is safe.

A rule of thumb if you have vertigo while breastfeeding, continue to breastfeed if you can, but only if it is safe to do so.

Having a new baby will make you so grateful for everything, like the fact that your cells didn't multiply and create quadruplets.

Baby Not Thriving?

Sometimes, babies don't thrive while being breastfed, for a number of reasons. None of those reasons are your fault. Babies like to narrate their own stories.

How can you help your baby if this is the case?

If your baby isn't gaining weight, your doctor or pediatrician is the first person to contact, and will be able to advise you on the best course of action. This might mean supplementing breastfeeding with formula, or if the baby is old enough, to start on solids. Remember, there are always people who can help.

Formula Feeding

There may be many reasons why formula feeding is the best option for you and your baby. At the end of the day, feeding your baby is about you and your mental and physical health and your baby, and that you are both healthy and happy.

There may be reasons that you cannot breastfeed:

- You have a health condition or take medication that means you can't breastfeed
- You are unable to produce enough breast milk for your baby
- Have experienced a type of trauma or surgery involving your breasts so you choose to formula feed
- There may not be a reason at all, you just choose to formula feed, and that is perfectly okay.

I've heard stories about breastfeeding mums struggling so badly with breastfeeding that it becomes an immense ball of stress. The mum is not happy. The baby is not happy. But when they change to formula feeding, they relax and enjoy their baby and bond with them adorning them will all the love that they feel.

Happy mum. Happy baby.

It is important to note that both breast milk and formula are complete foods for babies for their first 6 months.

Whether you are breastfeeding or formula feeding, ask yourself these questions:
- Is your baby growing?
- Is your baby healthy?
- If the answer is yes to both of these, you are doing a brilliant job of caring for bubs.

Crying Baby and Hearing Loss

Bloody Ménière's disease. If the vertigo isn't bad enough, you lose your hearing too. Gradually. If you do have hearing loss and worry about not hearing your baby for whatever reason, these are many baby monitors and wearable alerts available that will have a solution for you.

Crying and Hyperacusis

Now here's another level of losing your hearing that absolutely makes no sense at all. Hyperacusis - a disorder in loudness perception, in which a person has a reduced tolerance to sound, where ordinary noises are too loud, and or can cause discomfort or pain.

According to Pubmed, the triad of tinnitus, hyperacusis, and hearing loss remains an often-underdiagnosed combination of symptoms that causes physical, mental, and emotional distress for millions of patients. And here we are, Ménière's. We are very familiar with your hyperacusis.

Solutions: According to the Cleveland Clinic:
- Don't overprotect against sound. The more you protect your hearing, the more fear you invoke about the sounds, and will be overly sensitivity.
- Systematically expose yourself to the sound of crying
- Talk to a medical professional

Apparently, it's all tinnitus's fault!

Ah, babies! They're more than just adorable little creatures on whom you can blame your farts - Tina Fey

My story

I always laid on my side during a vertigo attack, even during my very first vertigo attack in 1996. When my baby needed feeding and my vertigo was being difficult, I would lay my baby safely beside me, and fed him or her, watching in my peripheral vision, while still staring at one flower on the wall paper to try and control my vertigo.

During my Ménière's struggle, I needed to feel like I had achieved something each day, for my mental health. I learned how important it was to keep things simple. This quote from La Leche League International, *The Womanly Art of Breastfeeding* speaks of this perfectly:

> *Accomplish one small thing a day. Maybe it's cleaning that counter, maybe it's writing one thank-you note or writing in your journal. Don't make the task too difficult.*

Advice from mums with Ménière's

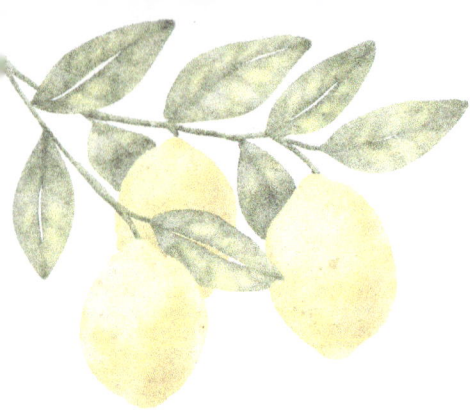

Dear Me,

Super Survival Mode!

* Three things I am thankful for.
* Do something I can achieve.
* Do something I love.
* Distract myself from Ménière's.

Every. Single. Day.

Love, Me

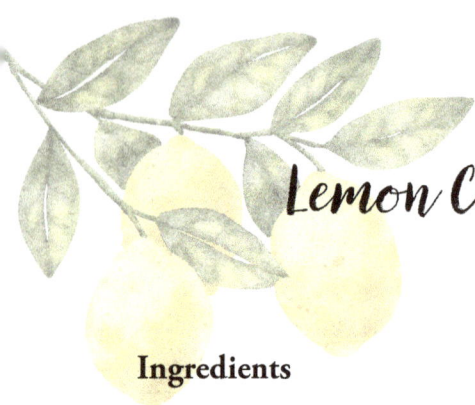

Lemon Coconut Slice

Ingredients

250g butter
430g (2 cups) caster sugar
4 eggs
225g (1 1/2 cups) plain flour
85g (1 cup) desiccated coconut
3 tsp finely grated lemon rind
60ml (1/4 cup) fresh lemon juice
Icing sugar, to dust

Directions

1. Preheat oven to 180ºC.
Line a 20 x 30cm (base measurement) slab pan with
non-stick baking paper.

2. Melt the butter in a saucepan over medium heat.
Remove from heat.
Stir in sugar.
Add eggs, 1 at a time, and stir until mixture is thick and glossy.

3. Sift the flour over the egg mixture and stir until well combined.
Stir in coconut, lemon rind and lemon juice.
Spread over base of prepared pan.

4. Bake for 30 minutes or until a skewer inserted into the
centre comes out clean.
Set aside in the pan to cool completely.

Cut into pieces.
Dust with icing sugar.

Notes (thoughts, photos, tweaks to recipe)

Ménière's and Motherhood
or the art of Aunty-hood, or looking after kids-hood

Whoa! You've made it through pregnancy, birth and babyhood with Ménière's. You are a rockstar! You have made it to legendary status! Well done! I can only say that because I am a Ménière's Mother Survivor. Three kids. Survivors of a mother with Ménière's!

My children are adults now. 28, 26 and 25 years old. All kind hearted with loads of empathy for others. I'm so proud of the people they have become!

Looking back at our lives from 1996 - 2004, Ménière's was an invisible beast always lurking, and from 2000, striking in clusters up to forty times throughout the year.

It had me scared. Some days I refused to drive. I would never go to the shops or the mall without my husband or my mum.

Looking back, my kids were my saving grace. The love they gave. They love I had for them and still have for them. The distraction from Ménière's they gave by us being together, playing games, having fun. Making wonderful memories.

All of those things dwarfed Ménière's. That's not to say it wasn't difficult at the time, because those vertigo attacks were horrendous.

I remember one time, being stuck on the floor of the toilet with violent vertigo, for three hours. I couldn't move my head, only to vomit into the toilet. So many times. By the time the vertigo had abated enough for me to move, I could only crawl along the floor to get to my bedroom. One of my kids thought I was playing and tried to climb onto my back for a ride. My husband carefully lifted my son off my back. I can only imagine how hard it was for him to watch me suffering. He wanted to help me to the bedroom but I said no. I needed to move by myself to make sure the violent vertigo wasn't going to hit again.

As a mum with Ménière's, way before I had any in depth

knowledge about Ménière's, or Internet, or social media, or knowing any women with Ménière's, I had to be super prepared all the time. I had a contingency plan in place for when the inevitable would happen, and I would be alone with my three kids with a violent vertigo attack. This is what I did with my three kids: My eldest had some responsibilities. If I went into a vertigo attack, I would tell him to:

- Phone Dad at work, or Grandy, and tell them I wasn't feeling well and needed them at home. He knew how to use the wall phone, and the phone numbers were written down for him.
- Play a video for his little sister and little brother, or play some games with them. He knew which foods and drink were okay for them to have when I couldn't get it for them

Within ten minutes, either my husband or my mum and dad were there to help me. And by that I meant looking after the kids, taking an enormous amount of stress from me, or cleaning out my vomit bowl. Regularly.

When my vertigo attack had ended after three or four hours, I would get up, wash my face and return to my family, even if I was exhausted from the vertigo attack.

These were the two essential strategies I had in place:

- Being prepared earlier with a plan for my eldest son to take over for a little bit, and
- To have my family rush home to help

These days I do have a mobile phone. It would be so easy to call a number of people on my contacts list to ask for help.

I realise how fortunate I was to have help, quickly, and I know that some of you don't have that back up. Is there someone who could help you if you don't have family. A neighbour? A friend? Another relative?

If I Couldn't Get Help

There was always the possibility that I could not get help. So I had to plan ahead:

- Have your Ménière's kit to grab - medication etc and take what you need to take as soon as you can.
- Let the kids know that you're not feeling well.
- Set boundaries - where they are allowed to go in the house.
- Lay down or rest in a spot in the house where you can all comfortably co-exist.
- Let the kids set up camp, make a fort, or make their own nest of blankets on the floor where you can see them.
- Have a special bag/suitcase filled with new toys, colouring, puzzles, drawing etc that only gets opened when you are unwell.
- If they are of reading age, they could read to you.
- Implement quiet time if they are old enough to understand.
- Let them watch TV or a movie, or play video games.
- Ask them to build something out of Lego.
- If there are older kids, ask them to help look after the younger ones.
- Keep reassuring your children that you will be okay.
- Accept that the house will become messy.
- Wait it out for either your vertigo to stop, or for help to come.

Whatever happens. You've got this. And remember, help will come soon, or the vertigo will stop soon. From my experience with children, they are very sympathetic and want to help you if they can. Children are a blessing! And they are blessed to have you as their mum.

When My Kids Were Older

Motherhood is messy and challenging, and crazy, and sleepless, and giving, and unbelievably beautiful.

I wish when my kids were young and I was struggling with the stress of having Ménière's to cope with on top of it, there were encouraging quotes around that normalized the difficulties all mums face with raising their children. I wouldn't have felt like a failure sometimes then. When I could go to mothers' groups when I was feeling okay, the other mums all seemed to have it together with their wonderful children, the mums with their ear to ear smiles who made life look easy.

Until a mum lost her temper at her child one day. She had had enough! And her tears fell. And then all the stories came out about kids and challenges and how they coped with the challenges. This was a mothers' group at its finest. When others listen and lift others up. It's okay. We all feel like that. We all have crappy days!

Hey, Mama. I see you stressed out, tired, touched out, stretched thin, irritable, snappy, imperfect, short-tempered, grumpy, crying, it's okay. Everybody has been there; it sucks, but you are good. You are a good mom, say it, believe it.

I never sent my kids to daycare or kindergarten, for a number of reasons. So, they were with me until they started at school. When I look back, I am so thankful that we could live on one wage at that time. Those precious early years with my kids are something I could never get back.

As my children journeyed through toddler-age, preschool-age, and until school-age, we had a routine for when I was unwell with vertigo. The routine stayed the same so that there was no confusion as to what to do. It would be my eldest calling my husband or my mum, who would come home as soon as they could.

You know, when I look back to when my kids were young, I know that I did have around forty episodes of vertigo a year, usually in clusters (I kept a journal of them so I could share it with my ENT, as well as time, duration, what I had eaten beforehand, what I had been doing etc), but I don't remember them clearly. I do however, remember the wonderful things my kids and I did at home together. Testament to the good outshining the bad. A saving grace.

Mother Guilt

"A mother's guilt is forever. The I-should-have-done-this or should-have-done-that will always be there. Learning to live with it is forever. Stop beating yourself up, accept it is a part of motherhood and keep being who you are. The mother guilt you feel is normal. Children don't even know the words 'mother's guilt'."

Although I don't remember every single violent vertigo attack I had when caring for my three children, mother guilt sneaks in sometimes. That little voice in my head saying I didn't do enough for my kids when they were young. Or that voice that says you're not the parent you should be with your education and teaching experience. Or that voice that said, if you didn't have Ménière's disease, would the personalities of my children have been different?

I didn't have mum guilt while I was journeying through their childhood, and me with Ménière's at the time. It's only in hindsight that these feelings emerged.

Things like:

- I didn't take them to Wiggles concerts, or other concerts that are tailored for children. They missed out on that joy.
- I didn't take them to the park to play when it was just us (in case I had a vertigo attack and couldn't get home)
- I didn't play rough with them (because I was scared it would set off a vertigo attack)
- I didn't make my babies laugh enough like other people do with shaking their heads and blowing raspberries on the baby's tummy (I was scared it would set off a vertigo attack)

My mother guilt is self-inflicted. I know it. I did the best I could at the time with a chronic, incurable, debilitating illness. I was in survival mode. I was in protection mode for my children, at all times.

"Breathe. Your kids need you, with your worries, and your laughs, and your fails, and you try-agains, your love, your showing up, that's what matters, breathe sweet mum."

Eventually, I learned to let the mother-guilt go. My kids were loved to the end of the universe and back and forever and a day. They were well fed. Clothed. Had a roof over their heads. They smiled and laughed. My husband was amazing with them, doing things with them that I couldn't.

And I thought one day, *how could they miss something they never knew existed - like Wiggles concerts.*

I chose not to live with chronic guilt that would lead to anxiety and depression and exhaustion or burnout. I was a better mum without those stacked on top of my Ménière's disease. Life is hard enough. You don't want to make your life harder.

Be Kind To Yourself. Always.

Life is not a competition. It's not about being a better mum than other mums. It's not about your kids being better than other kids.

Being a mum is about loving and supporting your children for who they are, warts and all, listening to them with care and empathy, and making sure that they know how loved they are.

Always.

> *"All your kids want is you. Not the fit mom, not the Pinterest mom, not the PTA mom, not every other mom you think you should be. All they want is you, so be the happiest you there ever was."*

Ménière's Mother Survival Kit

- Give yourself permission to take good care of yourself—self-care. Have you ever wondered why when you are flying and the oxygen masks come down, you are told to put yours on first, and then your child's.
- Be kind to yourself
- Have some me time
- Go for a walk
- Connect with nature, even if it is in the garden and admiring the miracles of flowers
- Don't compare yourself to others
- Accept that we are not perfect and make mistakes. Forgive yourself
- Pause in the hard moments. What are you feeling? And realise that other mums around the world feel that too, and struggle like you are. Then say some kind words to yourself.

> *"Successful mothers are not the ones that have never struggled. They are the ones that never give up, despite the struggles."*

You know what? When I ask my kids about what they remember about me when they were young, and I was in the midst of my worst Ménière's symptoms, they don't remember it.

'I've asked them many times—do you remember when I was sick and would lay on the bed for hours and hours, vomiting?'

They all would say no.

'I've asked them—do you remember standing beside my bed and holding my hand for a little while when I was unwell?'

None of them remember.

And I sigh a breath of relief.

I don't want them to remember how sick I was.

I am eternally thankful to my husband and my mum and dad who would come to care for the kids when I was terribly unwell.

It takes a village.

And you know what? I am the one with the terrible memories of wishing I could do more for my kids when they were young. Wishing I had happier memories of their early childhoods.

In 2004, when my kids were 8, 6 and 5, I had a full strength of gentamicin injected into my Ménière's ear.

It stopped the vertigo. For good. I now had the life I wanted to share with my kids. The one where I didn't have to worry about vertigo hitting at any moment. The one where I could drive at anytime, without fear. The one where I could do things with my kids, without having to have my husband or my parents with me, just in case vertigo came.

In hindsight, if I was planning on having a baby now with the better options of treatments for vertigo, and my vertigo was frequent and severe, I would have medical intervention before having a baby.

Life after my gentamicin injection in 2004 improved 1000%. It was an answered prayer. But I wouldn't choose gentamicin. There's a better option called **Endolymphatic Duct Blocking**. It stops vertigo, and leaves your hearing and balance intact. It's worth investigating if you have frequent Ménière's attacks.

Hope is a waking dream.

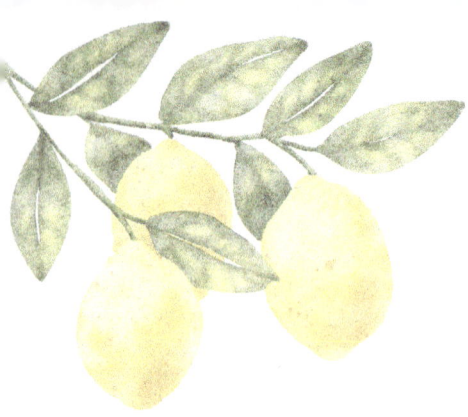

"A mother's love is more beautiful than any fresh flower."

—Debasish Mridha

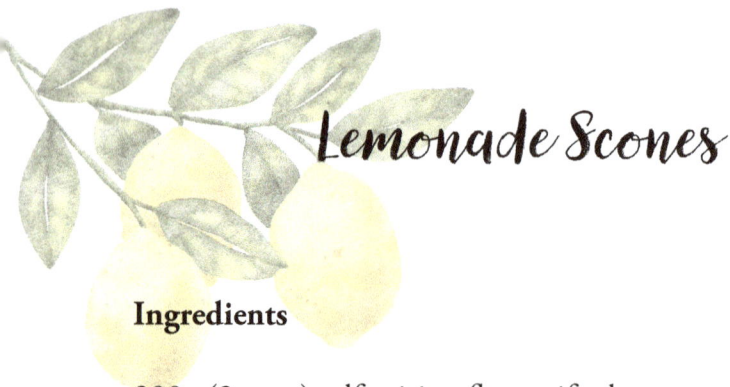

Lemonade Scones

Ingredients

300g (2 cups) self-raising flour, sifted
55g (1/4 cup) caster sugar
125ml (1/2 cup) thick cream
125ml (1/2 cup) lemonade
40ml (2 tbsp) milk
Lemon curd, to serve
Whipped cream, to serve

Directions

1. Preheat the oven to 220C.
Lightly grease a baking tray.

2. Place the flour, sugar and 1/2 teaspoon salt in a large bowl.
Add the cream and lemonade and mix to form a soft dough.
Turn out onto a lightly floured workbench and knead
lightly until combined.

3. Press the dough with your hands to a thickness of about 2cm.

4. Use a 6cm round cutter to cut out 8 scones, place on baking
tray and brush the tops with some milk.
Re-roll scraps to make a few extra scones.

5. Bake for 10-15 minutes until lightly browned.

6. Serve warm with lemon curd and whipped cream.

Notes (thoughts, photos, tweaks to recipe)

Ménière's, Perimenopause and Menopause

*And the beauty of a woman, with passing years
only grows! - Audrey Hepburn*

Just when you thought you had the hang of controlling your Ménière's symptoms the best you could with your monthly period, along comes perimenopause to stuff up your hormones again.

Lucky us.

On Ménière's Facebook pages, I often see women asking about their Ménière's symptoms with perimenopause, or menopause. They are trying to figure out whether what they are going through is normal when you have Ménière's.

Perimenopause and menopause are rarely talked about openly. It's one of those taboo topics of my mum's generation. Today though, more people and celebrities are starting to talk about it. All women go through it. It's a natural transition, marking the end of the reproductive years. Why try to hide that fact. It is nothing to be ashamed of. In fact, once you have your last period, it is an immense feeling of freedom. Of liberation. It's worthy of a celebration!

Perimenopause

Perimenopause means "around menopause". It's the stage of life leading up to your last period (Yahoo!) as your ovaries slow down.

It usually occurs between 45 - 55 years of age. For some women it can start in their mid-30s.

Perimenopause can last up to 4 - 6 years, on average. For some, it lasts up to ten years before menopause, and for others, only a year.

Perimenopause ends one year after your last period.

Be proud of how you show up every day,
feeling comfortable in your own skin,
being your magnificent you - Bonnie Marcus, author

Symptoms

The level of estrogen—the main female hormone—in your body rises and falls unevenly during perimenopause, causing irregular periods. They may come less often, sometimes even more often. They may be shorted or longer, your bleeding may be lighter or heavier than usual. Some months you may not get a period.

If you are one of the people whose hormones influence their Ménière's symptoms, this may cause your Ménière's to flare at certain times with the rise and fall of hormones. You can use the period tracker in this book to track your cycle and also add the MD symptoms you are experiencing.

Most females will experience symptoms of menopause, although 1 in 5 won't have any symptoms at all. Around 1 in every 5 females will have symptoms severe enough to affect their daily activities.

Symptoms of perimenopause may include, and please note: you may not experience all of these.

- Irregular periods
- Hot flashes/flushes
- Mood swings
- Low libido (sex drive)
- Headaches
- Insomnia and disrupted sleep
- Sore breasts
- Weight gain
- Vaginal dryness
- Tiredness and difficulty with concentration and memory
- Itchy or dry skin

- Sore muscles and joints
- Night sweats
- Brain fog
- Dizziness
- Heart palpitations
- Depression
- Anxiety
- Panic disorder
- Irritability
- Stress incontinence
- Digestive problems
- Bloating
- Muscle tension
- Body odor
- Hair loss
- Brittle nails
- Itchy skin
- Burning mouth
- Changes in taste
- Bleeding gums
- Tingling extremities
- Electric shocks
- Allergies

What a wild ride!

https://www.mbody.health/perimenopause/symptoms-treatment/why-you-should-track-the-34-symptoms-of-perimenopause

I see menopause as the start of the next fabulous phase of life as a woman. Now is a time to 'tune in' to our bodies and embrace this new chapter. If anything, I feel more myself and love my body more now, at 58 years old, than ever before – Kim Cattrall, actress

Research

I spent days in the bowels of the Internet trying to find research about Ménière's disease and perimenopause. As expected, there was hardly any research. I'm kinda thinking that we women just get on with life, even though the hard bits and hormonal changes and the extra level of Ménière's on top. We are our own tracking systems.

I did find this bit of information though:

> *A small 2013 study focusing on women with Ménière's showed that the number of vertigo episodes in premenopausal women was almost double that of postmenopausal, and additionally that 62.5% of the postmenopausal women reported having noticed an improvement in their symptoms after the menopause.*
>
> *https://www.menieres.org.uk/files/pdfs/Monaghan.pdf*

In my readings, I discovered that the incidence of BPPV (Benign Paroxysmal Positional Vertigo) increases with all women, Ménière's disease or not, during perimenopause and menopause, due to the increased hormonal fluctuations.

https://www.ncbi.nlm.nih.gov/pmc/articles/PMC7596253/

The Menopause & Post-menopause

> *Menopause. A pause while you reconsider men*
> *- Margaret Atwood, author*

Aaaaah! A sigh of relief. You have had your final period. You have not had period or spotting for 12 months.

Let the party begin! You are free from period pads and tampons and period undies and cramping and whatever else your body did unique to you in the lead-up to your period and whenever you had a period.

Except ...

During post-menopause, your body learns to function with low hormone levels, and symptoms caused by fluctuating hormones may become less troubling—or disappear altogether. Post-menopause also means your ovaries no longer release enough hormones to support a pregnancy.

According to an article published in 2019, there is a correlation between auditory-vestibular functions and estrogen levels in post-menopausal patients with Ménière's disease.

This study suggests that some women, who previously had no history of Ménière's disease, develop Ménière's disease post-menopausally.

Estrogen levels correlated with auditory and vestibular function in post-menopausal patients with MD. Low estrogen may be involved in the microcirculatory disturbance of the inner ear, affecting the occurrence and development of MD.

www.ncbi.nlm.nih.gov/pmc/articles/PMC6430344/

Having stated an increase in Ménière's disease symptoms post-menopause, I have also read in social media groups, that with some women, their Ménière's symptoms get easier to live with. Go figure.

But there is so much dependability here. For example:

- How long have they had Ménière's?
- Are they entering burnout phase?
- Are they on any medication post-menopausally?

One thing is certain, more research in this area is needed.

Is Perimenopause and Menopause Beating You Up?

If you are intolerant of the symptoms of perimenopause and menopause, and feel like it is just another terrible thing on top of your Ménière's to try and have to cope with, a conversation with your doctor is warranted. There are treatments that you can try that focus on relieving your signs and symptoms. Whether the treatments help with your unpredictable Ménière's symptoms, is something only you can discover. *https://www.webmd.com/menopause/guide-perimenopause*

My belief is that it's a privilege to get older. Not everybody gets to get older - Cameron Diaz

My story

I had quite a smooth ride through the hot flashes of perimenopause. I discovered afterward about the effect of Cipramil that I was taking for anxiety, inadvertently made my hot flashes way more tolerable.

Antidepressant medications are recommended as a first-line treatment for hot flashes in people who cannot take estrogen.

According to Harvard Health Publishing, *randomized trials have shown that certain antidepressants can reduce hot flashes by 50% or more. These include paroxetine (Paxil) and fluoxetine (Prozac) - SSRIs, and venlafaxine (Effexor). A randomized controlled trial has shown that citalopram (Celexa), cuts the frequency and severity of hot flashes by at least 50% in postmenopausal women. Results were published in the July 10, 2010, issue of the Journal of Clinical Oncology.*

Menopausal Hormone Therapy (MHT) can reduce menopausal symptoms as well. However, there is an added small risk of blood clots and breast cancer while taking it. It's not for everyone.

https://www.menopause.org.au/health-info/fact-sheets/what-is-menopausal-hormone-therapy-mht-and-is-it-safe

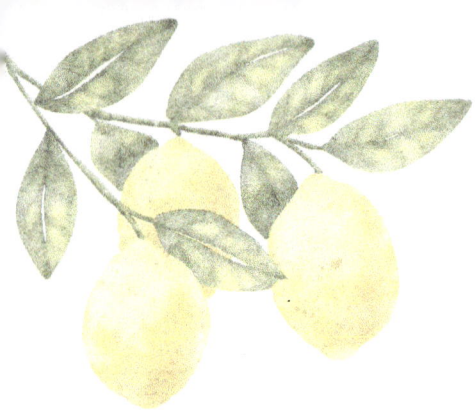

Dear Me,

Be *kind* to myself ...

intentionally,
extravagantly,
unconditionally.

Love, Me

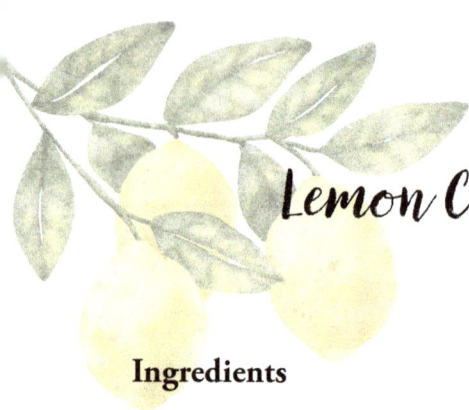

Lemon Custard Slice

Ingredients

3 x 250g packets Lemon Crisp biscuits
100g (2/3 cup) custard powder
55g (1/4 cup) caster sugar
1L (4 cups) milk
1 tbsp finely grated lemon rind
1 tbsp pure icing sugar

Directions

1. Grease a 3cm-deep, 20 x 30cm slice pan.
Line the base and 2 long sides with baking paper, allowing the paper to overhang the sides.

2. Place half the biscuits over the base of the prepared pan.

3. Place the custard powder and 125ml (1/2 cup) milk in a saucepan.
Whisk until smooth.
Pour in the remaining 3 1/2 cups milk.
Add the caster sugar then place the pan over medium heat.
Cook, stirring constantly, for 5 minutes or until the custard comes to the boil.
Cook, stirring, for 2 minutes or until thickened.
Stir in the lemon rind then remove pan from heat.
Cover the surface of the custard with plastic wrap.
Set aside for 30 minutes to cool slightly.

4. Pour the warm custard over the biscuits in the pan.
Top with another layer of biscuits.
Place in the fridge for 4 hours or until set.

5. Dust the top of the slice with icing sugar.
Use a sharp knife to cut the slice into even pieces,
using the shape of the biscuits as a guide. Serve.

Notes (thoughts, photos, tweaks to recipe)

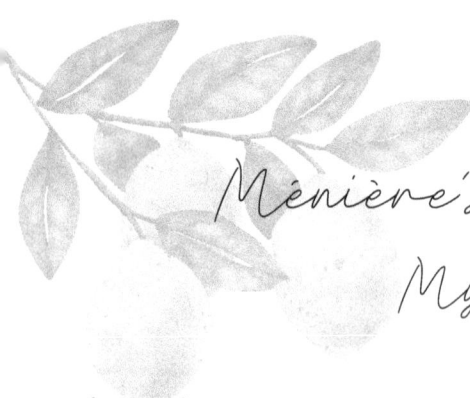

Ménière's and Work
My story

To tell your employer about your Ménière's, or not? Women and men alike battle with this question. Some inform their employer, some don't. You need to find out whether you are legally required to inform your employer about your condition?

During my teaching years, I always let my employers know about my Ménière's disease, even when I don't get vertigo anymore due to the gentamicin. It was for "just in case" vertigo decided to hit me again. I also gave them printed information to help them understand Ménière's a little more, and what to do if I did have a vertigo attack at school. One school principal was great, and sat and talked to me about it. When we had a change of principals, the new one put her hands up and said, 'I don't want to know about it.' My latest principal and head of secondary are very supportive.

Being a teacher is hard work. You have to be alert the entire time you are in class. There is no such thing as sown-time. Ménière's piled extra stress onto me with my hearing loss in my left ear, and the no direction of sound that went with it. I also feared having a vertigo attack in class and how I would cope with it, and who would look after my students as a drop of a hat.

Teaching secondary classes had less pressure, as there was always other teachers not on classes during different times of the day due to their class teaching timetable, and would be able to take my class if I had to leave immediately to the teachers' lounge to ride out my vertigo.

Nevertheless, planning ahead is a teacher *and* a Ménière's person superpower, and most probably your superpower too.

Ménière's In-class Vertigo Plan

If vertigo was to happen in class with 28 students, I would respond this way:

- Stay calm and focus on my breathing
- Send a pre-chosen student to administration to get help at once with the special card of information I had created (this had also been practised so they knew what to do), or call via the classroom phone and ask for immediate help
- Take Stemetil (vestibular suppressant and anti-nausea)
- Ensure students were safe in the task they were doing while sitting and staring at one spot, waiting for someone to arrive to supervise the class
- If a relief teacher was taking a while to come, I would then tell the class that I wasn't feeling well. I certainly did not want to scare them at all

Ménière's Work Survival Pack

I always wear my Ménière's medic ID and carry what I call my Ménière's Survival Pack with me. It's just like a large pencil case that fits inside my work backpack or handbag that has the below items:

- Stemetil (a vestibular suppressant that helps ease the vertigo)
- Vomit bag/s
- Water
- Face wipes
- Crackers (for nausea)
- Ginger (for nausea)
- A sweet in case of low blood sugar (jelly beans etc)
- List of phone numbers for either you to call for help, a friend, or a passerby
- An information card explaining Ménière's disease symptoms

And I always keep a change of clothes in the car, as well as toilet paper. Just in case.

Looking back at teaching while having Ménière's, I managed to not have a full violet vertigo at school. So thankful that my prayers were answered in that way. It seemed that they would occur however, waking me during middle of the night (and then I would go to school the next day), on the week-ends or evenings.

When my children were not of school age yet, I did a few relief teaching days. So when a teacher was away, I would get a call to come and take the class. The beauty of relief teaching was that if my Ménière's was in the lead up to a vertigo attack, and I would feel off balance, nauseous, unable to move my head much because it would make me more nauseous etc, I could say no to working that day.

One day though, I felt okay in the morning and throughout the day but when I got to the car to drive home, I started to spin. A slow spin. It was 2003, and fortunately I finally had a mobile phone to call my husband at work, who organised to come and drive me home. I had to wait an hour for him to arrive.

In 2004, I returned to teaching full time. I was terrified of having a vertigo attack at school. I made an appointment with my ENT who gave me prednisone to stop any impending attacks.

I clearly remember the first day I took the prednisone. It was like I never had Ménière's disease. My head was clear. My hearing was like it had returned to normal. I could do all sorts of things I hadn't been able to for six years or so. I was on cloud nine.

It was like I had found the cure for my Ménière's disease.

I went to school on the very first day of the school year. Full of confidence that my Ménière's was under control. And, before morning tea, while sitting on a chair reading to the students, vertigo started in a very. Slow. Spin.

I continued reading the book to the students, my hope of feeling normal plummeting like a wounded bird.

I also discovered that I couldn't sit or stand still. I had to moving all the time. I had lost my appetite, and then couldn't sleep.

On the third day of feeling like I had to get out of my skin, losing weight and no sleep, I rang my ENT who said I was allergic to the prednisone. I then had to start reducing the prednisone gradually. I went to my doctor, who gave me sleeping tablets.

That night I took the sleeping tablet, I still remember finally falling asleep. The feeling so welcoming. My body could finally rest and replenish.

Half way through the 10 week term my ENT put a grommet in my ear at his practise. He put a foaming anaesthetic into my ear canal and let it sit there for half an hour. While I was waiting, vertigo joined me in a slow spin. My ENT came into the room and suctioned out the anaesthetic, then popped in the grommet, and I went home, then off to school the next day, filled with hope that the grommet would stop my vertigo.

It didn't. The vertigo attacks continued in evenings and in the middle of the night.

It was time for a more invasive treatment. Gentamicin was next.

In 2004 I made the choice to destroy the balance cells in my left ear to stop the debilitating, violent vertigo. Th e vial of ototoxic gentamicin was now my hope. My ENT injected it into my middle ear through a grommet.

Imagine for one moment, having to make the choice about destroying your balance cells. Balance. *Yeah – that thing*. Something you never even think about. Your body just does it for you.

The day after the gentamicin injection, I woke up with bouncy vision. Every time I took a step, my whole world bounced up and down. I still had balance cells in my right ear, but destroying the balance cells in my left ear made my whole body balance precarious. It's called oscillopsia.

I had to slow down and relearn my new balance, and retaught myself how to walk with a damaged vestibular system. It was my new normal. I learned to use my eyesight as my guide for balance.

But compared to the unpredictable vertigo, the destruction to my vestibular system was an answered prayer.

It changed my life. It gave me my life back. With physical limitations. I was no longer spiralling down into the darkness of the Ménière's prison where there was no escape.

I returned to school after the June holidays with the hope that I wouldn't have any more vertigo.

I found it hard to trust that the gentamicin had worked.

I found it hard to allow myself to eat normally, instead of restricting my diet (which never worked anyway).

I found it hard to try to eat a more normal intake or salt.

The fear of eating normally and setting of a vertigo was very real.

But here I am in 2024. Still no vertigo. I am so very thankful for my answered prayer.

It doesn't mean that I was cured of Ménière's disease. It was that my vertigo was disabled. I still have hearing loss, tinnitus, imbalance and hyperacusis. But life was a thousand percent better without vertigo.

Your Ménière's Work Plan

Dear Me,

I must acknowledge my *limits*.
Don't *compare* myself to people
who don't have Ménière's disease.

And ... connect to *nature*.
It's good for the soul.

Love, Me

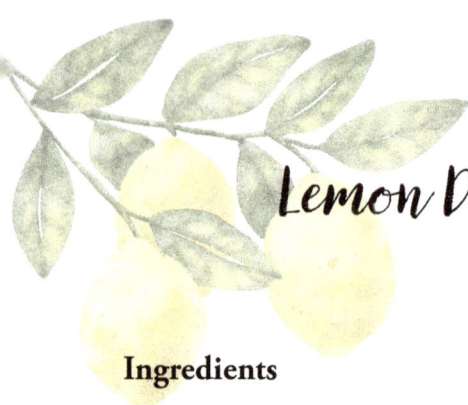

Lemon Delicious Pies

Ingredients

2 tbsp fresh lemon juice
2 tsp finely grated lemon rind
185ml (3/4 cup) milk
150g (1 cup) self-raising flour
35g (1/4 cup) custard powder
55g (1/4 cup) caster sugar
2 eggs, lightly whisked
100g butter, melted, cooled
1 tbsp bought lemon curd (or make your own)
Icing sugar, to dust

Directions

1. Place the milk, lemon juice and rind in a jug and whisk
to combine. Preheat the pie maker.

2. Sift flour, custard powder and caster sugar into a large bowl.
Make a well in the centre.
Pour the milk mixture, egg and melted butter into the well.
Use a metal spoon to stir until just combined.

3. Place 2 tablespoons of the mixture into each pie hole.
Place 1/2 teaspoon lemon curd into the centre of each pudding.
Top each pudding with another 2 tablespoonfuls of the mixture.
Close the lid and cook for 7 minutes or until just set.

4. Transfer puddings to a wire rack to cool.
Repeat with remaining mixture and curd.
Dust with icing sugar to serve.

Notes (thoughts, photos, tweaks to recipe)

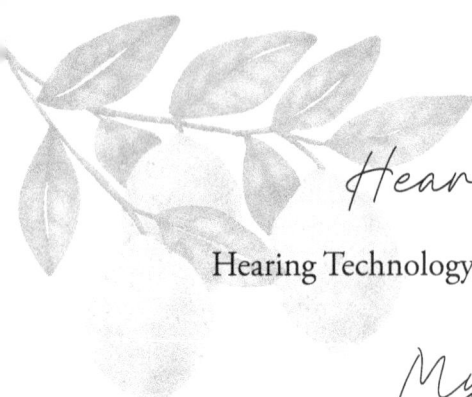

Hearing Loss

Hearing Technology and Hearing Gene Therapy

My story

I remember ironing school clothes when my youngest was in preschool. Tears were streaming down my face. He was five years old. My daughter was six and my eldest, another son was eight. It wasn't because my youngest was now going to school, it was because my hearing was getting worse and I was scared of never hearing my children's voices in the future.

I had to keep reminding myself that I still had hearing in my right ear. So that was something good to hold on to.

But still. Losing your hearing is terrifying. And absolutely a grieving process. Nobody asks to have Ménière's disease.

A few more years down the track, I had no word discrimination in my left ear. When I went for a hearing test, I could only work out two words. Going, and shopping. I think. Maybe. Or maybe it was that is was a bad hearing day for my MD? You know how our hearing fluctuates?

Do you ever do your own hearing scratch test?

My scratch test. A self-learned test I have been doing for 20 years with my Ménière's disease ear to see how much I could hear on any particular day. I scratch the "tragus", that little flap that sits in front of the ear canal. Sometimes I can hear the scratch sound. Other days not. Ménière's disease. Fluctuating hearing. One of the symptoms, until it doesn't fluctuate anymore. No hearing.

If you talk to people who have Ménière's disease, you will find that they have their own type of hearing test to determine how much they can hear on a particular day. Even Huey Lewis has his own hearing test, scratching the pillow/bed sheet to see what he could hear each morning. Then he gives it a rating out of 10.

And then there's the EarPod test. *My EarPod test.* A test I have regularly conducted in the 10 years before my cochlear implant, with hope that I had some hearing remaining, that I could still hear something. I would place the left EarPod in my Ménière's ear and stop the sound coming from the right EarPod then turn up to volume. Full Volume. The best I could hear at times was a short sharp SSH! Otherwise there was nothing. Just the sound of my disappointment.

Back to my audiologist. She said that a hearing aid for my MD ear would be of no benefit, as I wouldn't hear anything anyway. So I left with nothing.

The lesson I learned was, to get hearing tested earlier and grab a hearing aid that can also mask tinnitus earlier in the journey. It was too late for me.

Please don't make that mistake I made.

By the time I did get my first hearing aid, I had to have Cros hearing aids, where the left hearing aid would transfer the sound to my good hearing hear. I was excited for a bit because it meant I could hear whoever was on my left side. It also meant that my three kids wouldn't fight over who would walk on my right side, my good hearing ear.

And then, as good as the Cros hearing aid was, it was no good for me. In the classroom I needed direction of sound. The Cros hearing aid couldn't do that. Meanwhile, I had been talking to a friend, who also had Ménière's disease, and he had had a labyrinthectomy and a cochlear implant at the same time. He kept telling me how good the cochlear implant was and that I should get one.

Denial. Nah ... I don't need one.

When I finally decided to get a cochlear implant, it changed my life! I should have taken that step a long time ago, too.

Obviously I'm a slow learner in being kind to myself. I'm always putting myself last.

How is your hearing?

Do you need any technology to boost it?

If you are worried about how a hearing aid will look, or how a cochlear implant will look, or what other people will think, your ability to hear better and the improvement to your quality of life will blast judgemental people away! How dare they judge!

Nowadays, hearing aids are tiny, and the stigma that once came with having a hearing aid is next to none. Especially with more and more people needing help with hearing due to workplace hearing loss, listening to loud music, and COVID induced hearing loss.

Don't let others opinions of hearing aids let you miss out on sound that you deserve to hear.

One of the things that I love about my hair is that no one ever knew I had hearing aids, and now, they never know I have a cochlear implant. It's like my secret hearing superpower!

Good news developing in 2024 is gene therapy for hearing loss is restoring hearing. I'm looking forward to following the results.

Your story

_____

_____

_____

_____

_____

_____

_____

_____

_____

_____

_____

_____

_____

_____

_____

Tinnitus, I Hate You!

At the beach, every single time before 2020 ...

'It's so peaceful here,' my husband says.

I know he is talking about peace, as in no noise, except the ocean waves rolling in with a satisfactory sigh as the sand soaks up the salty water. I lift an eyebrow. I never had silence, or peace since Ménière's. With my FIVE LOUD NOISES OF TINNITUS!!!!!!!!!

I close my eyes and try to focus on just the ocean waves, whispering tales from the sea.

Nope. Try harder. Nope. Try harder. And there it is.

Habituation. Peace.

Have you ever ignored your tinnitus, and then someone talks about tinnitus and suddenly, you can hear your tinnitus again?

Like now. It's there isn't it? You can hear it clearly ... sorry.

I get annoyed when I try to tell someone about how TERRIBLY LOUD my tinnitus is, and they reply with, 'Oh, I have tinnitus too. It's so common. When it's really quiet, I can hear a little "ssssssssssss". You'll be fine!' I smile politely at them and hope I haven't inadvertently sent them the "looks could kill" look. They have no idea what the tinnitus of Ménière's is like.

Our tinnitus is caused by Ménière's hearing loss. It's the brain's way of trying to create a sound for the loss of sound input to your ear. So, let's go with a clicking or rushing or humming or pulsing or low-pitched ringing or high-pitched ringing or ssshssssshh or beeeeeeep.

Habituation

I think we all have a self-preserving feature built in to our brains that we can access with tinnitus. It's when you get so used to a noise in your environment (although tinnitus comes from your brain - it's trying to create sound for the loss of hearing input) that you stop noticing it. Like, it you live near a train line. When you first move in, you hear every train that goes past, but after a while, you don't notice the sound of the trains. It has a name, and is called habituation.

I stumbled upon ignoring my tinnitus when I first started writing novels. I would be so focussed on the writing that I didn't notice my tinnitus until I stopped writing. I was surprised when I learned it actually had a name. Habituation. Some people are so desperate to be able to ignore their tinnitus they actually pay someone to be their tinnitus coach. I completely understand, but also know that you don't need to pay someone to learn how to do it. There is an abundance of information on the Internet, plus there are free apps that help you as well.

Tinnibot is one such app. An award winning tinnitus app you can download onto your phone that helps you to habituate your tinnitus.

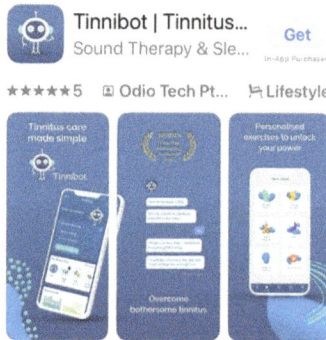

At the beach, every single time after the 9th January, 2020.

'It's so peaceful here,' my husband says.

I know he is talking about peace, as in no noise, except the ocean waves rolling in with a satisfactory sigh as the sand soaks up the salty water. I lift an eyebrow. 'I know,' I say, hearing the same peace that my husband can hear. Since having my cochlear implant, I have no tinnitus in my Ménière's ear when I am wearing the processor. When I take the processor off a night, I have one sound of tinnitus, that doesn't even rate on the list of annoying things.

Dear Me,

Be the *heroine*
of your *life*,
not the victim.

Love, Me

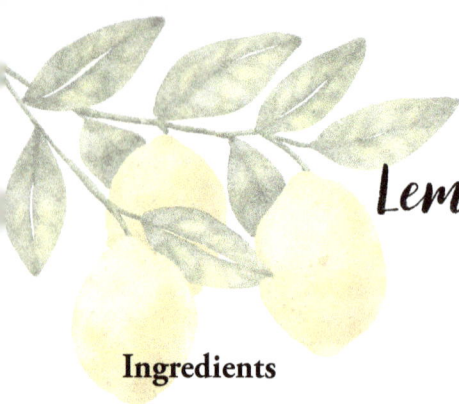

Lemon Tart

Ingredients

1 sheet frozen shortcrust pastry, thawed
1/2 cup caster sugar
1/2 cup lemon juice
1/2 cup cream
4 eggs
Lemon rind, finely grated
Icing sugar, for dusting
Thick cream, to serve

Directions

1. Preheat oven to 180C or 160C fan-forced.
Grease a 22cm pie dish.

2. Line prepared dish with pastry. Trim edges, using scraps to
patch any short sides.
Chill for 15 mins.

3. Line pastry with baking paper and fill with rice or
pastry weights.
Blind bake for 15 mins.
Remove paper and weights and bake for another 5 mins.
Cool in pan.

4. Mix together eggs, sugar, juice and rind and cream.
Pour into prepared tart shell.
Bake for 30-35 mins, until just set, but still a little wobbly.

Cool in pan.

5. Dust tart with icing sugar.
Serve in wedges topped with thick cream.

Notes (add a photo of your creation as well)

Got another headache, Batman?
How many times … it's a migraine!

The term used to describe a kind of migraine that mostly manifests as dizziness, is Vestibular Migraine (VM). Attacks can last anywhere from a few seconds to several days for certain patients, but they often linger for a few minutes or hours. The majority of patients report no headaches at all, but in around half of them, headaches or visual abnormalities (aura) follow or accompany the occurrence.

According to Meniere's.org.uk, *vestibular migraine is typically associated with nausea, vomiting, sweating, flushing, diarrhoea and visual changes such as blurring, flashing lights and difficulty focusing. Patients also report difficulty concentrating, finding bright lights and loud sounds uncomfortable and, most commonly, feel extreme tiredness and fatigue, needing to sleep.*

Significant hearing loss is associated with Ménière's disease.

There is a substantial correlation between migraine and Ménière's illness; almost 50% of individuals with the disorder have migraine symptoms at least once during an attack. Forty percent of people with Ménière's disease may have both diseases at the same time. Before beginning any harmful Ménière's treatment, patients with unexpected recurrences of their symptoms should always be evaluated for vestibular migraine.

Vestibular migraine is diagnosed on the patient's history. The presence of concurrent symptoms not expected in Ménière's disease such as blurred vision or sensitivity to light during attacks is often the key to the diagnosis.

The Journal of Neurology found a statistically significant association between hours-long attacks and Ménière's, but, with VM, vertigo could last for a matter of seconds to even several days.

https://www.ncbi.nlm.nih.gov/pmc/articles/PMC10025214/

Symptoms

- Severe, throbbing headache, usually on one side of the head
- Nausea and vomiting
- Sensitivity to light, smell and noise
- Vertigo (dizziness), usually lasting minutes to hours, but sometimes days
- Unsteadiness and loss of balance
- Sensitivity to motion
- Pressure in one or both ears
- Ringing

Treatment

Patients usually have one or more triggers, and treatment centres around managing the individual triggers. Triggers may be:

- Hormonal changes
- Hunger and dehydration
- Poor sleep - or too much
- Dietary triggers e.g. caffeine
- Stress and anxiety
- Lighting
- Stong odours
- Weather changes
- Smoking

If managing triggers is not effective, *lamotrigine* and *acetazolamide* may be more effective for the vertigo attacks than for headaches. Topiramate may be effective but requires more clinical data. Most treatment rests on the use of beta blockers, calcium channel blockers, tricyclic amines, and conservative measures like lifestyle and dietary modification. If available, a focused rehabilitation program directed toward migrainous vertigo, with attention paid to the additional mood and anxiety disorders, is likely to be helpful. *(Migraine-Associated Vertigo: Diagnosis and Treatment - Yoon-Hee Cha, M.D)*

My Go To
When Things Get Tough

The birdsong of the new day wakes me. If I had been sleeping on my good ear, I would never have heard it.

I'm thankful for that precious moment. It's been my survival mantra since battling through depression from the ferocious Ménière's disease.

Look for the small things that make me happy, no matter how small or insignificant they are to others.

It's been 29 years of Ménière's disease now. And even though I had my vertigo destroyed in 2004, it's been a helluva journey that had me on my knees pleading for mercy many times as I battled the violent, abhorrent vertigo that left me a shadow of myself, lost in the darkness of depression, trying to find me, my old happy, carefree, confident, successful self.

I've had to learn to practice self-compassion.

Don't compare my life to anyone else's.

That's a guarantee to make me spiral down. Just don't go there.

Be kind to myself.

This one takes practice. It's easier to do when I am in a place of acceptance of myself and my life and it's limitations. Nobody is perfect. I have to look for the small accomplishments each day, or the big ones, and celebrate them.

Give to others.

Giving to and helping others makes me feel happy. It's a way to keep focussing on the outside of me and not the inside of me and all my Ménière's symptoms.

Prayer

This is always my first go to. It changes my focus as I chat to God about things. Anything and everything. He understands perfectly what I am going through and what I am feeling. Prayer helps calm me and always brings about change to me or the circumstance. It makes me more thankful, and I can help others through prayer. It turns me from a worrier into a warrior! Prayer gives me hope, and I've seen miracles happen to me and others.

Your Go To When Things Get Tough

Ménière's and Being a Grandparent

At the time of writing this book my son and his wife are expecting their first baby. Our first grandchild.

My husband and I are both over the moon about a brand new person to love, and all the excitement and memories that will be made.

However, my husband and I had different reactions when we opened the box up with the pregnancy test. At first I thought it was a positive COVID test and thought, oh no! But then under the test were some baby clothes, and it all sunk in ... they are having a baby!

My husband teared up. He was thrilled beyond measure.

But for me, behind my smile and congratulations to my son and daughter-in-law, it bought back the memories of stress of when my kids were babies.

And then my brain started ...

What if... I am holding the baby and I fall over?

What if... I am holding the baby and I have a drop attack?

What if... what if... what if...

Thanks brain!

I had to stop my thoughts there, and change them around.

What if... I sit down while holding the baby ... safe.

I realised then, that when grandbubs is here, it will all work out. We will communicate and find solutions to ensure that the baby is safe, just like when I had my three babies.

Except this time, I don't have to worry about vertigo, and I have super enhanced hearing with my cochlear implant!

Life is going to be grand!

But what if I did get vertigo again? What would I do?

Realistically, I do need to be prepared for anything. Even if it's not my Ménière's that's not going to cause the problem.

Plan ahead:

- If you live alone and know that your Ménière's is building up and is a risk for spending time with your grandchildren, let the parents know and cancel the day.
- Have your Ménière's kit to grab - medication etc
- Let the grandkids know that you're not feeling well.
- Set boundaries - where they are allowed to go in the house.
- Contact the parents, or other family who could come and help or take over the care of the grandkids.
- Lay down or rest in a spot in the house where you can all comfortably co-exist.
- Let the grandkids set up camp, make a fort, or make their own nest of blankets on the floor where you can see them.
- Have a special bag/suitcase filled with some toys, colouring, puzzles, drawing etc that only gets opened when you are unwell.
- If they are of reading age, they could read to you.
- Implement quiet time if they are old enough to understand.
- Let them watch TV or a movie, or play video games.
- Ask them to build something out of Lego.
- If there are older kids, ask them to help look after the younger ones.
- Accept that the house will become messy.
- Wait it out for either your vertigo to stop, or for help to come.

Whatever happens. You've got this. From my experience with children, they are very sympathetic and want to help you if they can. Grandchildren are indeed a blessing! And they are blessed to have you.

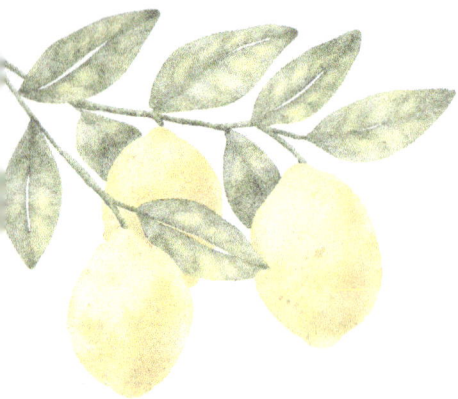

Dear Me,

It's okay, if all I did today
was to *survive*.

Love, Me

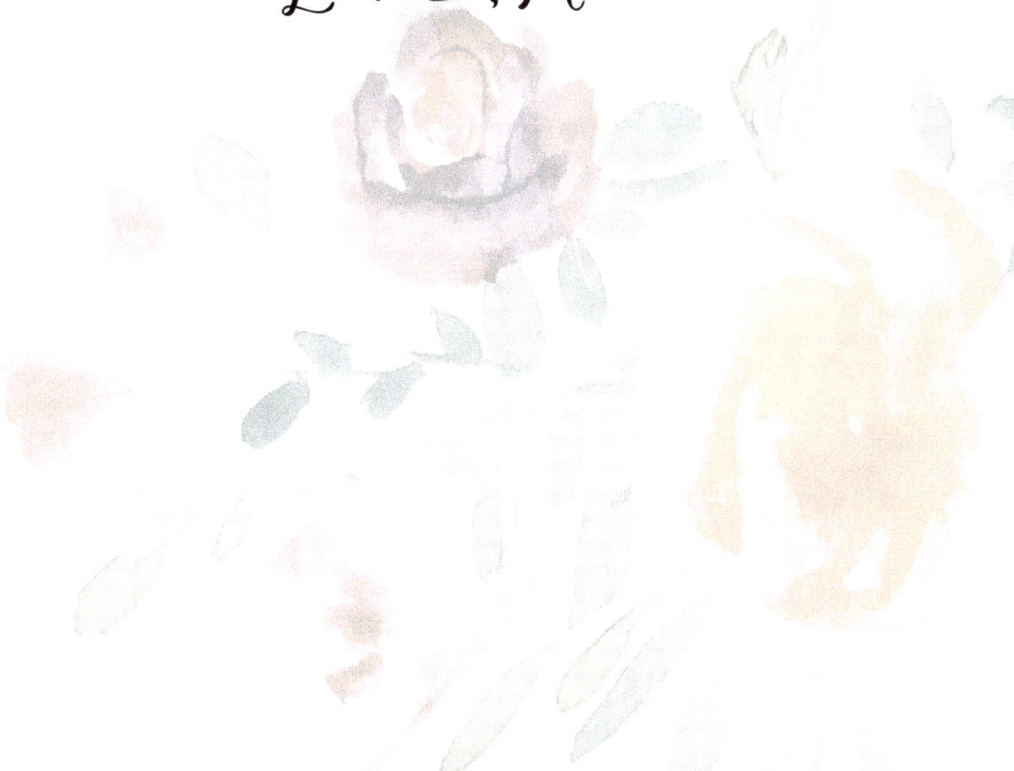

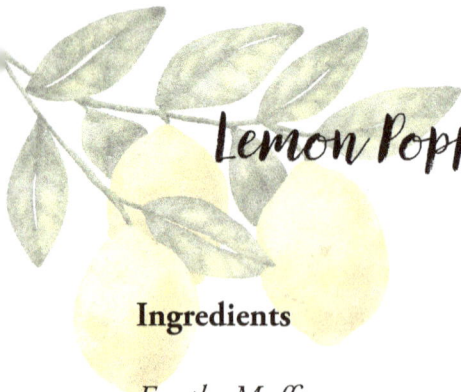

Lemon Poppy Seed Muffins

Ingredients

For the Muffins:
2¼ cups plain flour
2 teaspoons baking powder
¼ teaspoon baking soda
2 tablespoons poppy seeds
1 cup raw sugar
2 tablespoons lemon zest
1 cup whole milk Greek yogurt
⅓ cup full cream milk
1 tablespoon fresh lemon juice (15mL)
1 teaspoon vanilla extract (5mL)
½ cup unsalted butter melted
2 large eggs

For the Drizzles Icing:
1 cup powdered sugar (icing sugar)
2 tablespoons fresh lemon juice 30mL

Directions

Preheat oven to 425F.
Line a 12-cup muffin pan with paper liners.

For muffins
1. In a large bowl, sift together flour, baking powder, and baking soda.
Whisk in poppy seeds and salt.

2. In another large bowl, combine sugar and lemon zest. Working with your hands, rub zest into sugar until fully combined. Add yogurt, milk, melted butter, eggs, lemon juice, and vanilla.
Whisk until smooth.

3. Pour into flour mixture and fold just until combined. (Batter will be thick.)
Divide batter evenly among paper liners.

4. Bake for 15 to 17 minutes or until tops are golden brown and a toothpick inserted in the centre comes out with a few moist crumbs. Let muffins cool in pan for 10 minutes. Remove and finish cooling on a wire rack.

For glaze
6. In a small bowl, whisk together powdered sugar and lemon juice until smooth. Drizzle over cooled muffins.

Makes 12 muffins

Notes (thoughts, photos, tweaks to recipe)

Healing from The Grief and Trauma of Ménière's Disease

Having an incurable (for now) disease is life changing. Ménière's disease *may* cause broken dreams, broken careers, broken families, broken hearts, and sometimes broken spirits. And it may not. Or maybe you are just bruised by it. Whichever it is, no one comes out unscathed by it.

Ménière's is a grief journey

When you are diagnosed with Ménière's disease, you will go through the stages of grief, in any order, until you finally come to acceptance:

- Denial
- Anger
- Bargaining
- Depression and finally,
- Acceptance

There is no timescale for grief.

And there is no right or wrong way to feel.

The grief you feel is an emotional response to loss, or change to us that we have no control over. In my Ménière's journey, I didn't know grief was a thing, until I stumbled across it one day. I thought grief was something you went through when someone had died. When I educated myself about the stages of grief, it made perfect sense as to what I had been going through and the mourning of the loss of my former carefree life.

Trauma from Ménière's

Ménière's disease can cause trauma, depending on how severe and recurrent your symptoms are. Trauma is an emotional response to a terrible event. The event can come from the external environment, or a medical trauma - from within, like illnesses such as Ménière's disease. In fact, according to Psychology Today, people who live with chronic illness are at a greater risk of experience PTSD like symptoms (Post Traumatic Stress Disorder).

The good news is, healing from Ménière's trauma and grief is possible. Psychologists call it "post-traumatic growth". And that is about using adverse events such as chronic illnesses to make positive changes.

We are never left in a dark place with an illness. There is always a solution to lift you up. To heal. You will find it. Like I did. Although mine was accidentally.

I found healing in writing and in visual art. Writing with a character with Ménière's disease, and art filled with the swirls of vertigo. It was about getting my emotions and feelings and stuff I had suppressed with Ménière's disease, out of my system and onto paper and canvas mixes with a thousand tears. It was my own therapy.

And it was messy and beautiful and confronting and comforting.

And I was able to breathe deeply again.

And I was able to look back at the truck load of crap that Ménière's sent my way to my physical and mental self and know that I had survived. I had pushed back against the Ménière's monster instead of running away and hiding. I won.

I created new dreams. New goals.

A new way to look at the world around me and my place in it.

Healing is about acceptance of the situation. Acceptance of limitations. There is always a solution.

Creativity as a restorative tool

Art

> *Art washes away from the soul the dust*
> *of everyday life – Pablo Picasso*

For thousands of years, people have used the arts as a means of self-expression, communication, and healing. The practice of art therapy is based on the notion that mental health and healing can be promoted via artistic expression.

The goal of creating art is to utilize the creative process to assist you in exploring self-expression and, in doing so, find new ways to gain personal insight and develop new coping skills.

As you create art, you might examine your creations and the emotions they evoke, or you might not. Perhaps it's just the releasing of emotion that is enough. And it was enough for me. As you make more art, you might see recurrent themes and conflicts in your work that might be influencing your feelings, ideas, and actions.

Techniques for visual art you can use include:

- Doodling and scribbling
- Finger painting
- Colouring
- Working with clay
- Sculpting
- Collage
- Drawing
- Painting
- Photography
- And others. Don't let this list limit you.

> *Art enables us to find ourselves and*
> *lose ourselves at the same time – Thomas Merton*

Writing

Fill your paper with the breathings of your heart
-William Wordsworth

Writing is another way to enable healing from Ménière's disease. It's therapeutic and creative and expressive. You don't have to be a prolific writer, or even a writer to benefit from writing. All you need is a computer (or other technology - even voice recorder) or paper, pen and the motivation to write. Or buy a beautiful journal as a gift to yourself, as you write your way to personal growth. I find that even just buying the journal is uplifting to me (don't ask my husband about how many journals I have bought over the years, and not written in. It just gives me joy!)

As a teacher, I worry that the education system has put so much weight on the quality of writing, that the joy of writing has been sucked out of it. It's time to unlearn the heaviness of writing at school. Who cares if you can't spell? Who cares if the sentence doesn't make sense, as long as it is meaningful to you. It's not as if your writing is going to be broadcast across the globe for criticism. It's for your eyes. Your brain. Your heart.

You're not at school anymore.

Write.

And write some more.

Get that crappy Ménière's disease out of your system. It deserves the worst treatment with words that we can give it!

- Just write the words that want to spill out of you
- Journal
- Write a letter
- Poetry

- Free write
- Mind map (involves writing down Ménière's in the middle, and thinking of new and related ideas which radiate out from the centre. There are many mind map templates online to use)
- Mind tree (draw a tree or use a real tree. Add leaves to it with words on them. Ménière's words and feelings. Enjoy watching the leaves drop off, the Ménière's words returning to the earth never to be resurrected)
- Journal with photographs
- Timed journal entries (eg set timer for 10 or 15 minutes)
- Use writing prompts if you like (can be found online)
- Memories writing
- Song writing

A word after a word after a word is power
- Margaret Atwood

Writing tips

1. Don't hold back. This writing is for you first and foremost. Don't worry about grammar or spelling. Don't worry about what anyone else might think or whether it is well written or kind or fair.
2. Write honestly and openly
3. No detail too small; no feeling too large.
4. Don't edit.
5. Find the right place for you to write
6. Experiment with which writing type works for you.
7. Write freely and without judgment

One of the things I love about Ménière's social media groups, is that you can write about your symptoms, and express how it makes you feel. And I love all the support and care others give.

Other Creative Activities to Consider

Dance - uses body movement and dance, exploring different movements and rhythms. No dance skills or experience is needed (and besides, we women with Ménière's disease may have our own dance styles as we have a unique way with balance). Dance and movement may also be beneficial for strengthening balance pathways in the brain. If your balance has been affected by Ménière's, know your limitations with dance.

Drama - uses different types of drama and performance activities that gives you the space to share your thoughts and feelings. To add an extra level of interest. Record yourself to watch later and/or keep a drama log of expressing yourself about Ménière's disease. Talk to the camera. Release the words and feelings.

Music - involves exploring music and sound. Writing songs. Singing. Making music. Learning an instrument. You don't need to have any musical knowledge or experience. If you have lost your hearing, focus on the vibrations that music gives. One of my teaching friends is a music teacher. Her class is comprised of Deaf students. I asked her how she teaches music to Deaf students, and she said by vibration and beat vibration.

Added Bonus of Post-Traumatic Growth

A stunning added bonus to art and writing, or dance and drama and music, is that you may discover that you *can't hear your tinnitus*, or *you forget you have Ménière's disease,* even for a little while when you are engaged in creativity. When you realise that has happened to you, it's guaranteed to *make you smile*, and is a most welcome release from the prison of Ménière's.

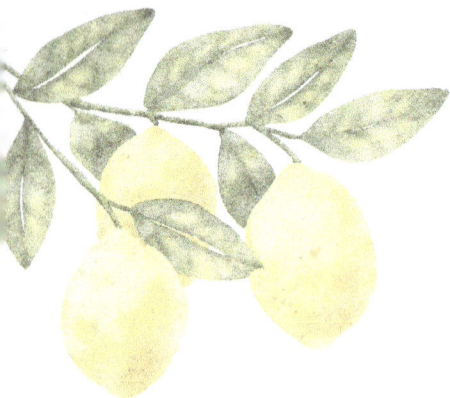

Dear Me,

When the cure
for Ménière's disease is found
~ and it will be ~
it will be because of
all of us,
working together.

Love, Me

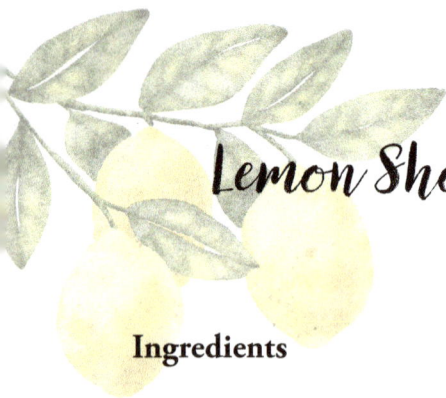

Lemon Shortbread Cookies

Ingredients

1 cup unsalted butter, room temperature
2/3 cup sugar
1 large egg yolk
1 tbsp lemon zest (from about 1 lemon)
1/2 tsp kosher salt
1/2 tsp pure vanilla extract
2 1/4 cups plain flour
1 large egg white
2 tbsp caster sugar and/or hundreds and thousands sprinkles

Directions

1. In the large bowl of a mixer, beat butter and granulated sugar on medium-high speed until fluffy and paler in color, about 3 minutes. Using a flexible spatula, scrape down sides of bowl. Mix in egg yolk, lemon zest, salt, and vanilla on medium speed until combined, about 30 seconds. Mix in flour on low speed until just combined, about 30 seconds.

2. Using spatula, scrape dough onto a sheet of plastic wrap. Pat to a disk, then tightly wrap. Refrigerate at least 2 hours.

3. Arrange racks in upper and lower thirds of oven; preheat to 300º F / 150º C.
Line 2 baking trays with baking paper. Place another large piece of baking paper on a work surface. Place unwrapped dough on baking paper, then top with another large piece of baking

paper. Using a rolling pin, roll dough 1cm thick. Using a round cookie cutter, cut out rounds and arrange on prepared sheets, spacing them apart.
Reroll scraps and cut out rounds from remaining dough.

4. In a small bowl, whisk egg white until frothy, about 30 seconds. Brush tops of rounds with egg white.
Sprinkle caster sugar or sprinkles over each.

5. Bake, rotating pans front to back and top to bottom halfway through, until cookies are firm to the touch, 25 to 30 minutes. Let cool on baking sheet 5 minutes, then transfer cookies to a wire rack and let cool completely.

Notes (thoughts, photos, tweaks to recipe)

Ménière's and Mindset

In one minute you can change your attitude and in
that minute you can change your entire day.
- Spencer Johnson

mindset

noun

a person's way of thinking and their opinions.

In the following pages, I'm going to touch briefly on Mindset. It's just scratching the surface, to be honest. If you are interested in Mindset, be sure to research online, purchase books or visit your library to do your own research.

Mindset is a big buzzword at the moment, developed by Stanford psychologist *Carol Dweck* way back in the 1970s, and her book was published in 2006. Growth Mindset was originally developed for students and education, but it has spilling over into the lives of, well, everyone.

It's based on the premise that, Mindsets can impact your reality - mindsets can impact your outcomes by determining the way you think, feel and even physiologically respond to some situations. And that Mindsets are not set in stone. You can change your mindset.

Although external influences have a significant influence on your perspective on looks and success, neural networks in the brain are malleable and can grow, evolve, and reorganize during the course of a person's existence. Any time in your life, you can create new neural connections, or mindsets, by pushing yourself with novel events and viewpoints.

The challenges posed by chronic illnesses, such a Ménière's disease are numerous. It may also seem to restrict us or alter the courses we take. A growth mindset accepts that, adjusts, and moves with the times. Simply put, receiving a diagnosis of an incurable, lifelong health condition presents a significant mental challenge.

Realizing that you may still lead a fulfilling life while suffering from a chronic illness can be a long-term process on the path to acceptance. That's all included in the growth attitude. You're probably going to be stuck feeling pretty terrible if you tell yourself that you're never going to get better, and that nothing will help.

On the other hand, your chances of feeling well increase if you accept that you can influence some things and that they will help you feel better. I don't intend to imply that you will heal yourself with it. However, you'll begin to feel more confident in yourself, grow happier, and possibly even experience way more good days than bad.

7 benefits of developing and nurturing your mindset

- It gives you are more **flexible attitude**. Change doesn't scare you as much and instead you embrace the challenge to find new ways in situations.
- Improving your **problem-solving and growth mindset** means that you have more faith in yourself. When you have faith in yourself, you are more likely to solve a problem. Your confidence in your ability to solve a problem means that you actually do it.
- When you believe that you can do anything with effort and hard work, it gives you the confidence to go for it and follow your dreams. **It gives you more drive**. How many times have you heard someone tell you that you can't do something, only to go for it because you were told that you can't? That's growth mindset!
- It **feeds your intellectual wellbeing**, one of the Six Pillars of Wellbeing. It is all about growing the mind and using the brain a little bit more. Developing and nurturing the growth mindset will improve intellectual wellbeing and make us feel better inside and out.

- A development mentality **makes us more open** since we're not anxious to come up short, or to celebrate our victories. As we create, we gotten to be more comfortable in ourselves which makes us feel more sure and open as well.
- It develops a **more optimistic mindset** as our mentality develops, so does our positive thinking. We begin to see the positives in circumstances, trying to find the silver lining and knowing that things aren't inactive and that's affirm.
- When your mentality is developing, it **creates opportunities** and you are more mindful of openings accessible to you And you believe that you can achieve those opportunities as well. our subconscious starts to notice opportunities which you may not have seen before.

Nurturing our Mindset

Embrace failure instead of fearing it. Look for the positives. What can you learn from the failure?

Keep learning to nurture growth mindset is a key element. Whether it is learning from new experiences and people, or failures, or learning anew skill. When we fail, we are actually learning. There is no growth without failure. What do you want to know more about? What are you passionate about? Keep an open mind, read, watch documentaries.

Don't be afraid to **ask questions**. There are no stupid questions. There's no disgrace in not knowing something. Learn from people around you. Ask questions about Ménière's disease. How can you help yourself? Research the research.

Remember, you are not Ménière's disease. You are more than your health. **Changing your narrative** from victim to *conqueror* will flip your attitude over to the positive.

Journal **the process**, so you can look back at how far you have come, acknowledging the hiccups along the way, and that you picked yourself up and kept going. Enjoy and embrace the challenges.

Developing your growth mindset

According to *Dweck* (2015), consistency is key.

1. Change your language
The language you use when faced with a challenge greatly affects how your brain will tackle that challenge. Negative language like "I'll never be able to do that," stalls information processing and can increase stress responses in the body. This causes the challenge to seem too big and complex for you to tackle, leading to stagnancy. Using positive language and praise when faced with a challenge, however, can improve wellbeing, self-confidence and better information processing. Ultimately, this helps strengthen our mental fitness and resilience.

2. Let go of perfectionism
Perfectionism alludes to the habit of holding yourself to an excessively high standard, and is often paired with overly critical self-talk. When we allow perfectionism to creep in, we often become easily frustrated when certain things don't go our way from the beginning.

Dweck (2015) states that when we only focus on our abilities in the "now" we completely cut off the possibility of our skills in the "yet". Instead, when we focus on information processing and problem solving with patience, hard work and learning, we experience steep skill and knowledge development.

3. Emphasise the learning journey
Intelligence is malleable and a curiosity for learning is essential for forming new neural pathways and expanding your intelligence. This is why, even when our hunger for learning diminishes, we persist in reflecting on how things work and why—developing our skills and knowledge even further.

4. Leave your ego at the door
Realising that your current abilities and knowledge are not adequate for the ahead challenge is sometimes a tough pill to swallow. In a fixed mindset, it leads us to quickly giving up and feeling bad or bitter for doing so.

It takes time and patience, but developing a growth mindset will greatly impact your overall wellbeing. From lowered stress to raised self-confidence, you'll start to approach situations with a healthy problem-solving attitude, rather than one of dread.

In a nutshell, growth mindset is focused on *possibility*.
- Be prepared to change your habits
- Appreciate the little things in life
- Routine and structure is important
- Make the choice to be positive
- Don't let Ménière's disease suffocate you. You are not your disease
- Acceptance of Ménière's comes first, and then you can grow

Changing your attitude towards failure, mistakes, and criticism by taking risks without fear.
1. Be kind to yourself
2. Read Books by People Who Have Overcome Adversity
3. Embrace Your Worst Fear
4. Challenge All Negative Thoughts
5. Use Your Imagination to Visualize Success

There are many books about Growth Mindset you can read from bookstores or libraries. It is worth noting, that if you have a hard to shift depression, Mindset may not work for you.

I know that when I was in my darkest place with Ménière's disease, I could not have worked on Mindset, because I was not in the right state of mind. However, when I finally when to my doctor and spoke about to her about how I was feeling, she started me on an anti-depressant, and that was enough to lift me out of the black pit, so I could slowly move forward to wellness, and a better outlook on my life. Being on anti-depressants didn't mean for life, it was just a tool I needed at the time. I was so very thankful for my doctor's understanding and care.

Cognitive Behaviour Therapy (CBT) and Ménière's

You know that voice in your head. That one that tells you, you aren't good enough. You'll fail. You'll never be good at something. You'll never feel happy again etc

It's lying to you!

Words have power. Power to change. Every single moment.

CBT is a type of talking therapy based on the idea that how you think and act affects how you feel. CBT helps you to recognise the patterns of thinking, and behaviour that causes you problems. From there, you will learn practical ways to learn or re-learn more helpful and healthy habits.

Basically, the aim is to challenge and break the habit of negative thinking. Negative and unhelpful thinking can manifest in different ways. You always assume the worst possible outcome, and you take everything personally, for example.

CBT focusses on goals and is specific to an individual. It doesn't look back over your past, it centres on solving current problems and has been around for many years.

According to *Iris Cahill Casiano, PhD*, if you are looking for ways you can do CBT on yourself, a cognitive-behavioral mindset is a great place to start. Here are couple of ways to start incorporating this mindset today:

Pay attention to thoughts. Often, thoughts happen so quickly we don't notice the kind of messages we tell ourselves. This is called our *self-talk*. Paying attention to our thoughts can help us start to notice if our self-talk is usually positive or negative.

Thoughts have a huge impact on how we feel. If our thoughts and self-talk tend to be more positive and supportive, we usually feel better about ourselves. But if our thoughts and self-talk tend to be unhelpful or negative, you guessed it: we might not feel that great about ourselves.

Just because we think something doesn't always mean it's true. Humans sometimes carry a negativity bias. This means that we often pay more attention to negative thoughts and experiences. Because of this, we might be more likely to believe negative self-talk about ourselves, even if it's not realistic or true.

Test your negative self-talk. Testing negative thoughts or self-talk with questions can help us see how accurate they are. Some questions might be:

- Do I have evidence for that negative self-talk?
- Do I have evidence against that negative self-talk?
- What are some ways those negative thoughts or messages might not be realistic?
- Are they 100% true, 100% of the time?

Embracing this CBT mindset might help us notice things about our thought process that we never paid attention to before. In turn, the more aware we are of these things, the more we can do to make positive changes!

Attitude and Ménière's

attitude

noun

1. a settled way of thinking or feeling about something.

Are attitude and mindset the same thing?

The quick answer is no.

A mindset is *a way of seeing the world*.

Attitude is *how you act in the world*.

So, basically attitude and mindset are not the same but at least are interrelated.

An attitude is a way we think and respond about something. It's our general outlook on life. Attitudes are performed through observation, interaction, and experience with the object, event, or person.

Attitudes are learned, but the good news is they can be changed.

People who are in your life often shape your attitude. Some attitudes can begin as early as birth while others start during your teenage years, when you are building a sense of self-identity.

According to *Sanju Pradeepa* from **Believe in Mind**, *the attitudes that you adopt at different times in your life will influence how you feel about yourself and what you do with your life.*

To develop a positive attitude:
1. *Stop Comparing Yourself to Others*
2. *Take Care of Yourself*
3. *Build Your Self-Confidence*
4. *Believe in Yourself*
5. *Think Before You Act*
6. *Smile More Often - smiling is one of the powerful ways to boost your mood and improve your health. It also makes you feel more confident and gives you an attractive appearance. Studies have shown that smiling can help to reduce stress and increase energy. It's also a sign that you are happy, content, and confident. You can start by smiling more often at work, in public places, and at home with your family. It doesn't take much effort to smile or laugh, so just start doing.*

In this chapter of the book, we have explored Mindset, CBT and Attitude. All three of these self-growth techniques require you to be consistent with working with them. You may find that one of them works, all of them work, or none of them work for you. If you are still struggling, and are finding that life is just abysmal and difficult, please see your doctor for either medication that will help you, just while you need it, or a therapist. Remember, there are people who can help you. You are never alone. And Ménière's mostly becomes less severe over time. There is a light at the end of the tunnel.

If you don't like something, change it.
If you can't change it, change your attitude.
- Maya Angelou

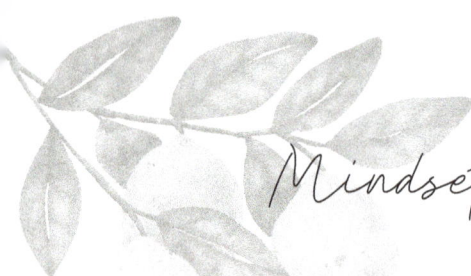

Mindset Examples

Mindset, Cognitive Behaviour Therapy and Attitude is a lot to take in. These examples may help you to understand those better, so you can utilise that way of thinking. A *fixed mindset* views talents, abilities, intelligence and creativity as *not changing*. A **growth mindset** believes those abilities and talents **can change** and **can be developed** with practice.

	Fixed Mindset	Growth Mindset
Challenges	Avoid challenges.	Embraces challenges.
Ability	Can't be changed.	Can be developed.
Effort	It's useless.	Path to success.
New information	Ignores.	Open to information.
Feedback	Ignores.	Learns from.
Ménière's	It will never improve.	Researchers *will* find a way to treat it successfully.
Vertigo	It's ruining my life. I can't work anymore.	It happens but I can be prepared. I'll let people know about it and what to do.
Tinnitus	I can hear it all the time. I hate it.	I will research it and try habituation so my brain tunes out of it. Perhaps a hearing aid can mask the sound.
Hearing Loss	I'll never hear again.	What technology will help me to hear again?
Balance	Nothing will help.	I'll find a specialist who can help.

Ménière's Fixed and Growth Mindset Examples		
Vestibular Rehabilitation	Fixed Mindset	Growth Mindset
Belief	You believe that Ménière's has changed your body so much it is beyond repair.	You believe that vestibular rehabilitation has helped you, and may prevent balance from getting worse.
Thinking	What's the use? Nothing will change. My balance won't get better.	I want to learn what I can to help my balance myself. And I will keep trying.
How the thought manifests in your behaviour	You watch TV instead of doing vestibular rehabilitation exercises.	You find a vestibular rehabilitation therapist who specialises in Ménière's disease.
The outcome	You spend less time moving and your balance deteriorates. You have to rely on others to get around.	The exercises improves your balance and you don't need to use a stick when you are walking.
How it makes you feel	You feel angry, frustrated and believe that this will be you for the rest of your life.	You are happy, pleased and have more confidence.

Ménière's and Anxiety

Do not anticipate trouble or worry about what may never happen.
Keep in the sunlight – Benjamin Franklin

Which comes first, the anxiety or the vertigo? Does vertigo cause anxiety, of does anxiety cause vertigo?

The American Journal of Otolaryngology, 2022, suggests that there is a high prevalence of anxiety and depression in patients with Ménière's disease. A study by *Dr. Foster Tochukwu Orjiin: The Influence of Psychological Factors in Ménière's Disease,* states there is a vicious circle of interaction between the somatic symptoms, especially vertigo, and the resultant emotional disturbances (anxiety), which in turn provokes the somatic symptoms. The quality of life is severely impacted by Ménière's disease and worse quality of life tends to occur in Ménière's patients with more severe vertigo.

https://www.ncbi.nlm.nih.gov/pmc/articles/PMC3952292/

Some people with Ménière's will suffer anxiety at the thought of having vertigo, while for others, the anxiety may come on when thinking of having vertigo at work or in public, or where they won't feel safe. While anxiety is a normal part of life, when it starts to impact the quality of your life, it can be part of an anxiety condition.

Anxiety feels like ...
Excessive fear, restlessness, tense wound-up and edgy, worrying, obsessive thinking, catastophising, panic attacks, hot and cold flushes, racing heart, tightening of the chest, quick breathing, difficulty breathing, headaches, pins and needles, trembling, gastrointestinal problems.

Does this sound familiar? I absolutely had anxiety with my Ménière's. It was my violent, debilitating and frequent vertigo attacks that caused it.

It's okay. The Ménière's family totally understand it. So, what can we do to sort out the which comes first, the vertigo or anxiety question. We can work on the anxious feelings. That we can control. And then we will see if our vertigo is not as frequent. Anxiety is the body's response to real or perceived danger, but there are immediate skills for coping with anxiety, and long term skills to keep anxiety at bay.

Anxiety Toolkit

Emergency Strategies
1. Question your thought pattern - are they true?
2. 4-7-8 breathing pattern. Inhale for 4, hold the breath for 7, and exhale for 8. Repeat two times only, otherwise you'll feel lightheaded. Also, if you have low blood pressure be cautious with this.
3. Use aromatherapy - lavender, chamomile or sandalwood.
4. Exercise. Talk a walk.
5. Grounding - 333 rule - name 3 things you can see, 3 sounds you can hear and 3 things you can touch.
6. Write down what's making you anxious. It gets it out of your head.
7. Count to 10 slowly.
8. Laugh.
9. Give anxiety a name and tell it to @*$! off!
10. Distract yourself.

Long Term Strategies
1. Identify your triggers.
2. Try therapy.
3. Keep a journal.
4. Stay active.
5. Limit alcohol and caffeine.

If you have tried and tried and tried to tame your vertigo without success, your doctor can help with anti-anxiety medication. It will be that helping hand up that enables you to cope better.

Ménière's and Self-Care

Self-care is how you take your power back - Lalah Delia

I t's vitally important that each of us makes time for self-care. Self-care that is meaningful, deliberate, and considerate benefits us. When we take genuine care of ourselves, we have the chance to learn more about who we are and replenish our energy before it runs out.

I have come to believe that caring for myself is not self indulgent.
Caring for myself is an act of survival - Audre Lorde

In the 2020's, it has been quoted that we live in extra-stressful times. And that is without having a chronic disease on top of everything else! Self-care has a number of important health benefits:

- Reduces stress (important for Ménière's)
- Improves resilience
- Improved happiness
- Reduces anxiety and depression
- Increases energy
- Reduces burnout

According to the World Health Organization, "self-care in important because it can help promote health, prevent disease, and help people better cope with illness."

Almost everything will work again if you
unplug it for a few minutes, including you - Anne Lamott

I'm just scratching the surface of self-care here. You can research it more thoroughly if you want to know more, including the seven different types of self-care. It's also important to remember that, despite its importance, self-care may not always feel natural or simple, particularly if you're not used to it. If this sounds like you, practise self-care in little steps at a time, and it will start to feel good over time. Self-care is not selfish.

There are days I drop words of comfort on myself like falling leaves and remember that it is enough to be taken care of by myself - Brian Andreas

Here's some self-care ideas for you and add your own:

Zone out for a bit	Chat to a friend	#SelfcareSunday
Clear clutter for 20 minutes	Cuddle with your furry friend	Watch something funny
Stay hydrated	Take a nap	Gratitude list
Focus on positivity	Take a warm bath	Catch up with friends
Journal	Listen to music	Pray
Walk in nature	Have a cup of tea	Catch some sunlight
Play a video game	Read a book	Listen to a podcast
Dance	Get a massage	Try a new hobby
Write	Create art	Take a stroll
Do something you enjoy	Go for a walk every day	Take a mental health day
Take a photo	Learn to say no	Social media off
Digital detox	Treat yourself	Compliment yourself
Tidy a living space	Pamper yourself	Timeout from kids
Gardening	Buy yourself flowers	Mindful breathing
Eat nourishing food	Declutter	Accept help
Go shopping	Play	Make something
Morning sunlight		

When we give ourselves compassion, we are opening our hearts in a way that can transform our lives - Kristin Neff

Ménière's and Burnout

Earlier in the book I wrote about the stages of Ménière's disease.

Stages of Ménière's Disease

Stage 1	Stage 2	Stage 3	Burnout
Vertigo sudden, unpredictable	Vertigo attacks less severe	Vertigo less frequent	No vertigo
Hearing loss comes and goes	Hearing loss and damage develops	Hearing loss becomes worse	Hearing loss profound
Tinnitus comes and goes	Tinnitus becomes worse	Tinnitus loud	Tinnitus multiple noises
Hearing and full ear sensation returns to normal between attacks	Ear fullness	Ear fullness	Ear fullness remains
	Periods of dormancy	Balance is affected	Balance affected

I have been in "burnout" since 2004, after having gentamicin injected into my middle ear to stop the violent, debilitating attacks of vertigo after nine years of living in that state of unpredictability.

So instead of a gradual loss of balance you will get as you go through the natural stages of Ménière's, I went to severe balance, then relearned my new balance with brain plasticity.

No more vertigo. I had my life back. Except, I still had tinnitus. My hearing loss was worse. And I still had ear fullness. But these I could live with. I couldn't live with the unpredictable vertigo anymore - 40+ attacks a year.

For me, burnout is a great place to be. I had been beaten down by Ménière's. But I have gotten back up again. I feel like a survivor. A warrior.

What's next, after burnout?

Rebuilding your life starts. Embracing the new you starts. And pursuing new goals starts. Wonderful days are ahead.

There are two parts of your new life. The emotional and the physical. With the emotional part, mindset will help you to move forward. You will need to give yourself time to grieve the loss of your old life. Who you once were and what you once did. And what's changed in your life. Life changes all the time for everyone. Without fear of vertigo, you will feel freed from the Ménière's prison , like you can breathe deeply again. You'll notice things around you with more vibrancy, more gratitude. You have fought so hard to get here. What an achievement!

Some of us will be able to go back to the career we loved, or find a more fulfilling career. *Possibilities*. I was able to go back to teaching. And I loved it more than I ever did as I thought I would never be able to teach again.

Be kind and gentle to yourself. *Honour your past*. This will help with acceptance of your post-Ménière's self. Plan new things. Add fun. Figure out what works for you now. What's best for you. And don't compare yourself to anyone else. You'll need to acknowledge that you have physical limitations with hearing and balance. Tinnitus will still be your companion but you can learn to habituate it, if you haven't already. Step up and find hearing technology that is suitable for you. You'll be surprised how much confidence hearing gives you.

Step up and do balance rehabilitation. You'll be surprised how much it helps you. But know your limitations. Focus on what you can do, not what you can't do.

The way I am looking at the hearing loss and balance of Ménière's, is that we are ahead of the curve, as all people have difficulty with hearing and balance as they age. We'll be better at it because we've had lots of practise!

And finally, be patient with yourself. You are a work in progress. Enjoy your vertigo free life! Celebrate it once a year!

Ménière's and Vestibular Rehabilitation

In 2004, nine years after my Ménière's started, I made a conscious decision to have my balance cells destroyed. I couldn't do the horrendous, unpredictable, debilitating, violent, torturous, four-five hours of insane vertiginous spinning and nausea and vomiting and staring at one focus spot on the wall for the entire four-five hours anymore. I was more than done. I didn't want to be here anymore. So when my ENT offered to inject gentamicin into my middle ear to kill off the balance cells, halting the vertigo, I didn't think twice.

The next day I had bouncy vision when I walked. It has a term – oscillopsia. Oscillopsia is a vision problem in which objects seem to jump, jiggle, or vibrate when they're actually still. It stems from a problem with the alignment of your eyes, or with the systems in your brain and inner ears that control your body alignment and balance. It was a side effect of having my balance cells destroyed. It was a good sign that the gentamicin was working, my ENT had said.

Three weeks later I was back teaching full-time, learning to trust that I wouldn't have anymore vertigo attacks. Since 2004, I have been vertigo free. So thankful for God's mercy and grace.

Nowadays, I would not opt for Gentamicin, I would opt for the Endolymphatic Duct Blocking. It doesn't damage your hearing or balance.

In 2019, before my Cochlear Implant, my surgeon insisted that I do balance rehabilitation. The therapist talked me through some vestibular exercises for neuroplasticity – the brain relearning balance. I cannot express how happy I am to get these exercises. They will help me no end.

Except, each of the exercises make me feel insanely nauseous.

I blow a controlled breath through my lips. I'm an expert at it.

'Do you want to stop?' she asks me during each exercise.

'No,' I say. 'I can do this.' And I get through to the end.

For four weeks, I did daily balance exercises at home. At first, the exercises made me extremely nauseous, but the more I did the exercises, the less nauseous I felt, until they exercises didn't make me nauseous anymore. At the start of vestibular rehabilitation, I could only do two heel-to-toe steps and then fall over. By the end of rehabilitation, I could do 100+ steps of heel-to-toe without falling over. It was that good!

What is Vestibular Rehabilitation?

When there is injury to, or an imbalance between the right and left vestibular organs (balancing organs) in the inner ear, the brain can reduce dizziness sensations by using a process called vestibular compensation.

In essence, the brain learns to maintain balance by depending more on alternate signals from the eyes, ankles, legs, and neck in order to counteract the disorienting impulses from the inner ears.

Vestibular rehabilitation improves balance and mobility, and can make a marked improvement in someone's quality of life improving their confidence. It's especially effective with PPPD (Persistent Postural-Perceptual Dizziness - symptoms such as unsteadiness, dizziness, or non-vertiginous dizziness, which are present most days f and exacerbated by positions such as sitting upright, standing, or walking and visually complex stimuli.

Types of exercises
- Head movement exercises
- Throwing a ball and catching it
- Walking
- Gaze stabilisation exercises

Meniere's.org.uk has an excellent PDF you can download.

https://www.menieres.org.uk/files/pdfs/balance-retraining-2012.pdf

Alternative Treatments and Natural Supplements

*** This information is for educational purposes only and must not replace professional medical advice. Consult with a healthcare provider before implementing any changes to your health regime.

Ménière's disease is frustrating (understatement, I know!). Some prescription medicines work for some, but not others. Prescription medicine did not work for me. Alternative treatments didn't work for me as I tried to slay the Ménière's beast with my sword of knowledge and research and trialling of integrative medicines. I believe that it comes down to the cause of our Meniere's, which researchers agree, there is no one cause of Meniere's, and that's why finding successful treatment is so frustrating.

Whether you have tried prescription medicines and have been left disappointed with results, or that you prefer not to take prescription medicines, we inevitably conduct our own research to find something that will help our Ménière's disease in our quest to eradicate our symptoms. Because complementary therapy treats the full body rather than just a portion of it, it is sometimes referred to as a holistic approach. While there might not be a full recovery from these therapies, they might help manage your symptoms and improve your day-to-day functioning.

** It is crucial that you let your doctor or other healthcare provider know about any new treatments you plan to start in case of reactions to other medications you may be on. I might also add to be careful not to overdose yourself on any natural supplements. My mum unknowingly did this and suffered from tingling and numbness in her hands and legs, and brain fog.

** **It is important to note that the nature of the fluctuating of Ménière's symptoms may lead you to think that the treatment is working. So it would be suggested that you keep on the treatment until your symptoms return again. This would indicate the treatment isn't right for your Meniere's.**

** **You also need to beware of the power of the mind, the placebo effect— your brain can convince your body a fake treatment is the real thing. For a while anyway.**

Alternative Treatments found in a Ninja Internet Search and also known from discussion in Ménière's groups. **Not advocating, just listing:**

Grommet
Upper Cervical
TMJ
Acupuncture
Chiropractic
Atlas Orthogonal Technique
Massage
Osteopathy
Reflexology
Cranio-sacral Therapy
Homeopathy
Hypnotherapy
Cannaboids
Herbal medicine
Meditation
Mindfulness
Sound Therapy
Essential Oils
Tai Chi (balance rehabilitation)
And others ...

Every alternative treatment/therapy/herbal medicine has a unique treatment plan, so you should think about which one or ones will be most effective for you. Do a thorough Internet research like a worried mother hen who does better research than the police.

Before you start the therapy, make sure you understand everything completely. Try no more than one new therapy at a time, and give it some time to work. Consider switching to a different treatment if you find that it isn't helping.

It is crucial that you let your doctor or other healthcare provider know about any new treatments you plan to start. You can employ complementary therapies in addition to prescription therapy, but before beginning any treatment, **be sure to discuss your Ménière's illness and any medications you are currently taking with the therapist.**

You should learn as much as you can about the therapy and the provider, including the therapy's credentials, track record, and reputation. You should also inquire about what happens during the session, who can benefit from the therapy, its costs, and its benefits and drawbacks.

Websites

I have listed the following websites that may help you in your search.

- *https://dizziness-and-balance.com/disorders/menieres/treatment/ alt.html*
- Ménière's.org: *https://menieres.org/alternative-metaphysical/ menieres-disease-herb al-treatments-supplements/*
- Ménière's org UK: *https://www.menieres.org.uk/information-and-support/treat ment-and-management/complementary-therapy*
- VEDA: *https://vestibular.org/article/diagnosis-treatment/ treatments/complementary-alter native-medicine/supplements/*
- **John of Ohio Treatment (known as a shotgun treatment combination of several vitamins, food additives, herbals,

and homeopathic substance) *https://menieres.org/forums/ database/joh-john-of-ohio-regimen-for-menieres-disease- details.6/* You can download a PDF of the treatment plan.

Before you embark on your quest to find what helps you, ask yourself these questions. They may guide you to what treatment you need to try.

1. *What do you know about what happened prior to the onset of your Ménière's symptoms?* It may point you in the direction of what complementary therapy/medicine to try. For instance, if it started after a virus, or COVID, your body would most probably be reacting to the inflammatory effects of the virus. If you were in an accident prior and had whiplash, perhaps you need to look at Atlas Orthogonal Technique. A recent head injury, middle or inner ear infection, or a more serious condition may be at the root cause of the symptoms. Please seek medical attention for a proper diagnosis before you start your search for finding something that alleviates your symptoms.

2. *Have you tried prescription medicine for Meniere's, which has been rigorously trialled and tested for effectiveness and safety?*

3. *Have you been diagnosed with Ménière's disease by an ENT,* after testing for Ménière's to rule out other causes of your Ménière's like symptoms?

4. *Is the alternative treatment suitable for you and your other medical conditions?* **Consult with your doctor first.**

Daily Ménière's Journal

Keep a Daily Ménière's Journal (FREE downloadable PDF *https:// myshadowmenieres.files.wordpress.com/2021/12/daily-detailed-3- month-menieres-disease-journal-december-2021.pdf)*– Is it stress that exacerbates your symptoms. Are you able to remove what causes the stress? Is it a food sensitivity, like gluten? Use the Daily Ménière's Journal to list the treatments you are trialling so you can keep track of the symptoms to know whether what you are doing or taking is helping.

Due to the sheer volume of herbal medicines available, *lack of long term safety on some herbal supplements, and also undeclared add-inns (possible contaminants) in the herbal medicines that you have no idea is in there (do you really know what you are taking?), and scam sites claiming to cure Ménière's (be careful),* I will leave you to research alternative medicines in depth. Ensure claims are backed up by science where possible, and check reviews online as to the quality of the company, the product and the processing of the product.

For your interest, here are some commonly used herbal medicines used across the world for Ménière's disease—**not advocating, just listing:**

Lipoflavinoids
Vinpocetine
Valerian
Ginger Root
Gingko Biloba
CBD Oil
Pycnogenal
Ginger
Echinacea
Lysine
Ebselen (which is used in SPI-1005)
And not herbal, but oats - SPC-Flakes

***Always check with your doctor or pharmacist that the supplements don't interact with other medications you take.
*** No medicinal content in this book, regardless of date, should ever be used as a substitute for direct medical advice from your doctor or other qualified clinician.

Dear Me,

Sometimes the best thing you can do is

not to think,
not wonder,
not imagine, not obsess.

Just *breathe* and have *faith*
that everything *will work out.*

Love, Me

Ménière's Management Plan

I love it when Menierians share their MD management plan. It encourages us to create our own. Here's one that a practitioner created for their patient:

For Emergencies only:
• For Vertigo - Cinnarizine
• For Anxiety - Lorazepam
• For Nausea - Ondansetron (Zofran)

Maintenance: *Daily Ménière's Journal, plus*
No drugs
Salt reduction

Some exercises to try:
• Pilates
• Walking at various speeds
• Zumba
• Freestyle swimming
• Aerobic style exercises
• Walking on foam while watching tv
• Toe touches
• Ballroom dancing
• Standing on foam with eyes shut for 60 seconds

You might read through the list and think, *oh, I cannot survive without my maintenance medication*, or *ballroom dancing will set off a vertigo attack*. You need to remember this was created for an individual person and their Ménière's story. We are all different.

But what the essence of this list is, that it is addressing not only the *now symptoms* of Ménière's, the *in-between symptoms*, but also *balance rehabilitation exercises* to help the brain maintain balance.

It is proactive and gives you a sense of control over Ménière's, boosting your ability to deal with the pressure of living with an unpredictable disease. Write your own management plan. It will have incredible mental benefits and give a boost to your coping ability.

Your Ménière's Management Plan

For Emergencies only:
• For Vertigo

• For Anxiety

• For Nausea

Maintenance: *Daily Ménière's Journal, plus*

Some exercises to try:

Ménière's and Mind Wanderings

THE HIPPOCRATIC OATH of doctors:

I will prevent disease whenever I can, for prevention is preferable to cure.

The problem with Ménière's disease is that there is not *one* cause of the disease, but many. This has been acknowledged by Ménière's researchers the world over. There is no *one* medication that will stop it. So if you hear a company claiming that their medication will stop all vertigo of Ménière's disease, or cure Ménière's disease, be wary.

If only we had a crystal ball to look into our future self to see what happened to us to cause our disease, so we could avoid that incident, that virus, those foods. Genetics is a different ball game, one that is currently being researched by world leading Ménière's disease expert, *Professor Jose Antonio Lopez-Escamez*, at the University of Sydney and Kolling Institute in Australia. He has established the Ménière's Disease Neuroscience Laboratory at the Kolling Institute where he is investigating the cellular and molecular basis of the disease, as well as the genetic factors contributing to severe tinnitus. His team are also working to identify molecular targets for personalised treatment. *https://kollinginstitute.org.au/world-leading-menieres-disease-expert-joins-the-kolling*.

I sometimes imagine what my life would be like *if* I didn't have head trauma from the softball training incident. Or *if* I didn't have the herpes virus in my body, caused by chicken pox (my mum's sisters decided that when one cousin had the chicken pox, we would all have a sleep over so we all got it), or from my mother's family, who still insist on giving you a kiss, even though they have a cold sore on their lips. *Run. Run away. Fast!* I am the only one who has Ménière's disease out of my twenty-seven cousins. I was the only one with a head trauma from sport. So it makes sense that treatment for my Meniere's would be different to someone's whose is genetic, or someone's whose is caused by COVID, or another virus.

On a side note, rumination about *what if* aggravates anxiety and depression. I have learned the hard way not to look back.

The problem with Ménière's disease is, instead of proactive prevention (because most of the time you don't know you will end up with it, unless it is genetic), we present with the symptoms, are diagnosed, and then live in a world of reactive medications and treatments.

Recently, in a Ménière's group page, I read about someone who had caught the flu and colds and other viruses that were impacting their Ménière's symptoms. But they were adamant that if they stuck to a healthy food regime and herbal supplements that it would halt the attacks. It wasn't working. Then someone said, have you tried antibiotics proven to help with that flu? Immediately a herbal practitioner chimed in, saying to add more supplements, and also said that, "not everyone can tolerate them".

Likewise, on another Ménière's site, someone had sudden hearing loss. Again they had tried a long list of herbal treatments, to no avail. Then someone said, have you tried Prednisone? And their hearing returned.

How long should you keep pursuing herbals, anti-virals, prescription medicines, alternative treatments, or following the advise of someone telling you that your stress is causing it, spending precious time to de-stress, only to find that isn't your trigger, all the while losing your hard earned money, confidence and livelihood and friends. Your quality of life. And yourself, wishing for the old you back. The you before Ménière's disease?

That was me. Searching and not finding. Hemorrhaging money.

At what point do you say enough is enough of the suffering, and choose a procedure that *will* stop the vertigo and stop your hearing and balance loss.

If there was a procedure that could stop your disease, stop your vertigo, your hearing loss, and retain your balance, would you do it?

I totally understand wanting to find a cure using herbal treatments and what nature has to heal us. I tried all of those things early in my Ménière's journey, plus alternative treatments, like sound therapy, acupuncture etc. (it's a loooong list). I believe that God has given us everything we need on the earth. As well as intelligence to create medications from plants. Many of the medications created in the past century came from naturally occurring molecules in nature, which can be found in a variety of sources, such as fungi, bacteria, and plants. Now, *drug discovery relies on the collaborative efforts of researchers including chemists, biologists, and physicians. Chemists build molecules that may eventually become drugs while biologists investigate the relevant molecules that cause diseases. Together, scientists select drug targets in the form of large biomolecules ... then search for molecules that will disrupt the protein or kill the cells causing the problems ...*

https://sitn.hms.harvard.edu/flash/2011/where-does-medicine-come-from/

Ménière's disease. No cause. No cure. Some doctors say, "You have Ménière's disease, I can't do anything for you." They are forgetting to add "intervention". This is what we *can* do for you.

And while we wait for the holy grail of Ménière's disease treatment, research is ongoing around the world. I applaud, with a standing ovation, those researchers who have not given up the fight for us. Ménière's must be a frustrating disease to research!

As I write this, I know that an implantable device is going ahead for trials that give you feedback on ions in your inner ear and will tell you of an impending vertigo attack via an app, so you can activate the release of those problem-causing ions in your inner ear to stop the attack (researchers at Curtin University – *Dr Daniel Brown* and Macquarie University – *Dr Mohsen Asadniaye Fard Jahromi*).

There is hope.

And researchers in genetics will give rise to correcting the gene causing the problem if your MD is familial.

There is hope.

But these interventions will be some time off as they go through rigorous testing and safety. Do you wait for years and years and years for these to become available, losing more hearing and balance, or do you take action to stop your attacks to preserve your hearing and balance and quality of life now?

I took action back in 2004 to stop my horrendous vertigo after nine years, after I tried alternative medicines and therapies and prescription medicines. They didn't help. The gentamicin damaged more of my hearing and took my balance, which I relearned with rehabilitation, and a cochlear implant gave me back my hearing. I never regret it though. It was what was available at the time. And it gave me back my life. An answered prayer. And for that I am forever thankful.

If I had a choice of intervention now though, in 2024, it would be the Endolymphatic Sac Duct Blockage that preserves your hearing and your balance and stops the vertigo.

I love that we have choices. And this chapter is purely my thoughts on paper. Simply food for thought. You may agree wholeheartedly or disagree with a passion. One thing is certain, you need to make the right choice for you, the severity of your vertigo, your circumstances and your beliefs.

A cure, or successful treatments for Ménière's disease are on my list of prayers.

It will come.

A hero is an ordinary individual who finds the strength to persevere and endure in spite of overwhelming obstacles - Christopher Reeve

Advocate for yourself. Be your own hero.

Your Letters

What would you say in a letter to Ménière's?

Dear Ménière's,

Letter to yourself *before* Ménière's disease

Dear Me,

Letter to yourself *while having* Ménière's Disease

Dear Me,

Letter to your *future self* **without** Ménière's disease

Dear Me,

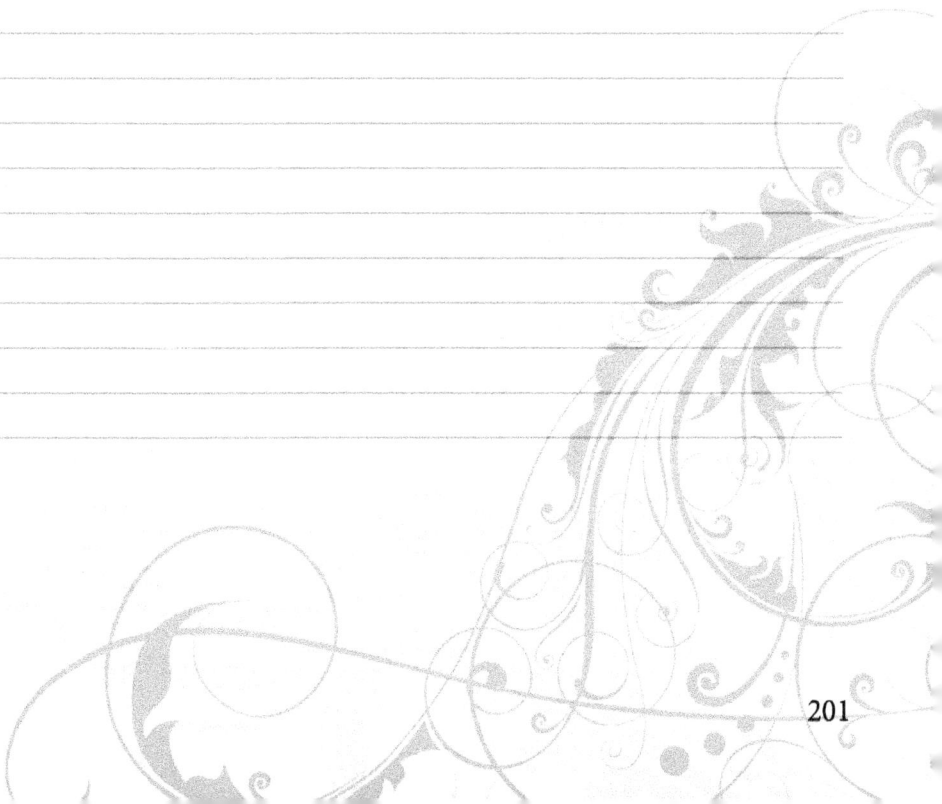

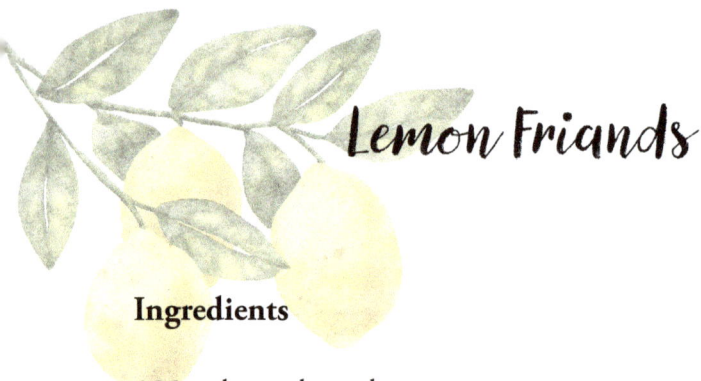

Lemon Friands

Ingredients

120g almond meal
60g plain flour
190g unsalted butter
1 1/3 cups (200g) icing sugar, plus extra to dust
5 egg whites
Grated zest of 1 lemon

Directions

1. Preparing the friand pan
Preheat the oven to 180°C.
Melt the butter and use a little to grease a 12-hole friand pan.
Dust with a little flour, shaking out excess.

2. Sift the flour and sugar into a large bowl, then stir in
the almond meal.

3. Place egg whites in a small bowl and lightly froth with a fork.
Add to dry ingredients with melted butter and zest, stirring
until completely combined. Fill each friand hole two-thirds full.

4. Bake for 25-35 minutes until golden and a skewer inserted
in the centre comes out clean.

5. Remove from the oven, leave in the pan for 5 minutes,
then turn out onto a wire rack to cool completely.

6. Dust with icing sugar just before serving.

Notes (thoughts, photos, tweaks to recipe)

Faith

Ménière's and Faith

Faith

complete trust or confidence in someone

I love this quote:
> *What gives me the most hope every day is God's grace; knowing that his grace is going to give me the strength for whatever I face, knowing that nothing is a surprise to God - Rick Warren*

My family never went to church. My family never discussed God, or Jesus, or prayed. But here I was, the introverted girl with the quiet God and Jesus belief who grew into the introverted teenager with the quiet God and Jesus belief who grew into the woman with the quiet God and Jesus belief and a strong faith.

Never in my life would I have predicted that I needed that believe in God and Jesus to carry me through the storm of Ménière's disease, and my life, in general.

God whispers. Listen to Him.

❧

One Monday I watched some fearless people build their hang gliders at the top of a cliff for hours. And then finally, there was a woman in her 40s, full of confidence ready to jump off the cliff to catch the uplift and fly. She looked like she had jumped off the cliff with her hang glider wings a hundred times.

She lined up her hang glider near the edge of the cliff and spotted her direction of take-off.

I thought how brave!

How inspiring!

It reminded me of having faith in God, taking a leap of faith, and trusting God that the outcome would be good.

Then I watched her falter more times than I could count, each time right before take-off. Fighting the fear. Trying to step out of her comfort zone, but being unable to.

Then other hang gliders gathered around her and talked her through take off.

Words of encouragement.

Support.

It reminded me of when people are struggling, and how God sends the helpers. Remember that person who helped you once?

I like to call them God rescue packages, and glitters. They come in the form of people, but also as animals, nature, words from the bible. He also blesses you with talents you had no idea your possessed, to open and use at the appointed time.

God is so gracious.

Loving.

Kind.

As I watched the woman struggling to take flight, it got me thinking, can you have trust without faith? Are they independent of each other? Or do they work together? Or does one build the other?

And then it reminded me of my life. A–B. Easy right. I have a plan. I am at A, and I know how to get to B.

Simple.

Done.

When I was little I wanted to be Batman.

This was not God's plan.

By the time I was nine, I wanted to be a nun because I loved God so much.

This was also not God's plan!

When I attended primary and high school, my favourite parts of the day were morning tea, lunch time, going home and school holidays.

Teaching could never have been in God's plan...

But guess what. I became a teacher, even though I was that student in high school who was way too introverted to answer questions in class, and told my friend sitting next to me the answers, who then gave the answer to the class, and the teacher thought *she* was really smart. I would just look down and smile meekly. Outside of school, sport, music and art were my passions. Every afternoon. Every weekend.

After I accepted the mission of teaching I was married, have children (before I lost all my patience on kids at school) and teach until retirement.

Simple.

Clear cut.

No bumps.

No obstacles.

Life's a breeze.

A straight line from A to B!

My life in reality is a messy scribble on paper and in my mind—teaching, and throw in facial paralysis at twenty-seven years of age (Bell's Palsy), Ménière's disease from twenty-nine (violent vertigo, tinnitus, deafness, ear fullness), three children (a blessing), deep dark depression due to Ménière's disease, in a very bad place trying to find the missing pieces of me, thinking of ending my life, balance cells destroyed to stop the vertigo (answered prayer), relearning to walk using my sight for balance, becoming an author (never expected that in a million years!), having a cochlear implant, relearning to hear again (answered prayer), being a research subject at the University of Queensland's mind and brain centre to help people with Ménière's disease, twice.

You know the seasons of life? I have an added extra. The tumultuous storm with my Ménière's disease.

But through it all, when I look back, God was there. Watching over me. Even though it didn't feel like it at the time.

Often times God demonstrates His faithfulness in adversity by providing for us what we need to survive. He does not change our painful circumstances. He sustains us through them - Charles Stanley

You know what really gets me about that quote? It's talking about God's faithfulness to us, not the other way around. It just makes me go WOW!

In my life journey , I've learned from God's plan:
- *Don't judge others.* You don't know what they have been through or are going through.
- *God is always there even when you think he is not,* or you start to believe the lies that you are unworthy, or you must be so bad that you deserve all of this.
- *Trust* in his plan.
- His plan is *far more exciting* offering your opportunities beyond you imagination – eg interviews, invitations interstate, zoom with USA, holidays etc.
- *He sends gifts to open when you least expect it,* or when you are in a low place you think you can't get out of – bible verses, people, the beauty of nature, writing to escape from my reality of no balance, extremely loud tinnitus, deafness, *The Colour Of Broken,* long listed twice to be made into a movie.
- He speaks to you. *God whispers.* He sends dreams, like in 1999 when I was in a very bad and dark place with Ménière's ... in the dream, I was sitting at a church where Darlene Zschech (my cousin) was preaching and she called me up to speak on stage—instant speaking in public fear filled me—all I remember thinking was that God would give me the right words to speak—I walked to the stage to speak to a couple of hundred people and said that God sees you and what you are going through. He sees your entire life from beginning to end. This is where you are right now and it will get better. I shared my dream with a friend who was going through a difficult time with chronic fatigue, even though it was a message for me and my suffering. My friend wrote me a letter a year later, saying what I shared with her changed her path and he chronic fatigue was gone. Twenty-one years later 2020,

Darlene asked to interview me about my Ménière's journey and faith on Instagram live. Again, I thought, God will give me the words. I did prepare beforehand as Darlene had sent me the questions she might ask, which took some pressure off. And this time, it wasn't around 200 people I would be speaking to like in a church, she had 440, 000 followers.

God speaks in the silence of the heart - Mother Teresa

In 2022, four weeks before my father died, I had a dream that someone had arrived at the place where I was, which was outside on a road. The day was lovely. I put my arm around that person and said, 'I'm glad you're here, he doesn't have much earth time left.'

On the 22nd June, 2022, Dad was admitted to hospital. The doctors where going to adjust his medications to take the load off his heart so he would feel better. In the afternoon, Mum and I left the hospital to go home to get some clothes for him. As I was walking out of the hospital rooms, I heard in my mind, *go back and talk to your father.* Three times. But I ignored it. I knew exactly why I had to go back and talk to my dad. It was to have a conversation with him about God and Jesus, before it was too late. And I ignored it. I wrestled with my lack of courage to go back and speak with my dad all afternoon and into the night. As I lay in bed that night, I made the decision to go to see Dad at the hospital first thing in the morning, regardless of the visiting times.

But I was so worried I was going to be late to see him and had lost the opportunity that, I called my eldest son and asked him to ring Grampy and talk to him and pray with him.

As I was driving to the hospital, I asked God to put the right words in my mouth to talk to Dad about Him and his Son, and rehearsed in the car how to talk to Dad about God and Jesus and whether he believed in them and to talk about heaven. In the car my conversation with Dad was so smooth and wonderful.

It wasn't the first time that I had talked to my Dad about what he believed because I thought that his time was near for quite a few years. The last time I talked about God to my dad, my kids were there. Me, Dad and my three kids. I asked Dad whether he believed in God. He shook his head and said, 'I don't know what I believe.'

My eldest son handed him his favourite leather bound bible and said, 'Grampy, start reading from Mark.' But he never did.

And that was it.

When I arrived at Dad's hospital bed he was sitting up with all the beeps and alarms you hear in Emergency. He was smiling at me.

On my way, walking to his bed I was stressing about how to bring up the conversation I needed to have.

'You're here early,' he said.

'Mum told me your phone wasn't working.'

'Sometimes it does but other times it doesn't. Declan called me this morning and he was saying something but I couldn't hear him.' I thought, that was him praying for Dad and with Dad.

Dad didn't hear it.

'Let me look at your phone,' I said.

Dad handed me the phone. I sat down and started to look at it, but I was bursting with 'I need to talk with you words'.

'Dad. I'm going to heaven and I want to see you there when I get there. I need to know if you believe in God?' These words fell out of my mouth like they had been in a tumble dryer. So much for the smooth delivery I had practised in the car.

He nodded his head. 'Yes,' he said.

'And Jesus? Do you believe in Jesus?'

Dad nodded his head. 'Yes. I always have. But nothing is going to happen to me,' he said.

In my mind I heard, *yes it is.*

'And,' I said, 'you know when you pass away, you are not alone. The angels are there waiting for you.'

Dad nodded. And I knew I had said enough.

That afternoon, while Dad was waiting for a transfer to another hospital to potentially get a heart pacemaker, Mum and I were hit with a shared trauma.

Dad lifted his left hand to his head and said, 'I've got a pain in my head.' And then his eyes rolled back and the alarms went off. There was a rush of frantic activity around dad while the nurses worked on him, and mum and I were quickly ushered out of the room. Despite all their efforts, Dad's last chapter on earth had ended.

Mum and I were brought back into his room. I went on one side of Dad, and mum the other, and I prayed for Dad. And I prayed for my mum and for God's grace and love and comfort for her.

And then came the shock. The numbness. The sobbing. Me witnessing my beautiful mum screaming out at my dad to speak to her. My mum trying to climb onto his bed and pleading for him to take her with him ... a few days later, while climbing over our mini dachshund dog gate in our house, I heard God say, 'Why are you looking for signs of your dad? He is with Me and I have given your peace. And that is enough.' God whispers. It was true. God had filled me with peace about Dad's passing.

God's timing is always right.
Trust Him.

John 3:36: Whoever believes in the Son has eternal life

When I was in the midst of my violent, frequent vertigo attacks in my thirties, I struggled with "why me?". My wings felt like they had been clipped and I was grounded, not allowed to reach my potential or dreams.

Each time that I lay staring at the wall, spinning, wherever I was, even on the floor in the toilet for four hours because I couldn't be moved during the vertigo, I felt like I had no more 'what'. What was my life supposed to be? What was my career or job supposed to be? I couldn't work. What was my purpose?

It was just me. With nothing. Like a brain with awareness and a decommissioned body experiencing the internal lie that I was spinning, and yet in reality, my physical body wasn't. I was capable of absolutely nothing. I felt like a nothing. I was a nothing.

I could move my arms and legs, but I couldn't move my head. If I did, it was catastrophic. The spinning was impossibly more terrifying. So, I did the only thing I could—I stared at one spot on a wall for three to four hours, wherever I was, spinning, exhausted from the spinning, the nausea, the vomiting. The only thing left I had was my mind. Me and my mind. Alone. Experiencing a philosophical existential crisis way before it became a thing.

As I rode the out of control spinning merry-go-round, I would imagine myself in heaven, bowing down before God, singing songs of praise with the angels, freed from Ménière's disease with perfect hearing again. It was the only thing that kept me going besides Jeremiah 29:11:

"For I know the plans I have for you," declares the Lord,
"plans to prosper you and not to harm you,
plans to give you hope and a future."

The only thing I had left as my life was stripped bare, was my true-identity. I am a child of God.

As brutal as having Ménière's disease is, I am blessed. It is my constant reminder of God's love for me. It made me realise that small things are big things. It made me search for my blessings and to count them, even in the midst of the darkness when I was on my hands and knees trying to find the pieces of my life that had been lost. Without God shining a pinpoint of Light in my internal darkness, I wouldn't be here.

There's a lot more to my journey, but the beautiful thing is, God answered my prayers, in His way, and in His timing, and he threw in unexpected blessings as well.

God answers prayers in a way that will blow your mind. He is extravagant!

According to Ephesians 1, *we have been blessed with every spiritual blessing; we have been chosen, adopted, redeemed, forgiven, grace-lavished and unconditionally loved and accepted. We are pure, blameless and forgiven. We have received the hope of spending eternity with God. When we are in Christ, these aspects of our identity can never be altered by what we do.*

Blessed. Lavished. Forgiven.

I love those words. Verbs. Our identity is in a God of action, of redeeming grace, a loving God who gave his only Son for us.

I am not a "what". I am a "who".

Did I pray for healing in my Ménière's journey? Absolutely. Sooo many times. *And* heard a "No!" And so I accepted it. But God didn't answer my prayer according to what I wanted. He had something way better than I could ever have imagined.

I had to learn trust.

Do I look at my Ménière's as a punishment? No. I look at my Ménière's as a reminder of God's love for me. How many times He guided me out of the darkness. How many times Jesus carried me through the impossibly difficult days. How many times He has given me the feeling of peace, when I should have been a ball of messy, ugly stress.

He never leaves us. God's got this. Trust Him in the storm. Thank Him in all kinds of unpredictable days. He sends us God whispers and unexpected rescue packages. Look back at your journey and you will see them.

That afternoon of watching people take leaps of faith off the cliff with hang gliding, I caught a plane back to Brisbane with my husband. I remember looking down at the earth from way above and beyond the clouds, and was caught by how we are invisible from a distance. It's like we don't even exist.

But to God, we are everything. We matter. We belong.

We are loved. He sees us. And He hears us.

And He *will* deliver us from our troubles.

And it will be more magnificent than you can imagine!

Dear Me,

Jeremiah 29:11

"For I know the *plans* I have for you," says the Lord. "They are plans for *good* and not for disaster, to give you a *future* and a *hope*."

Love, Me

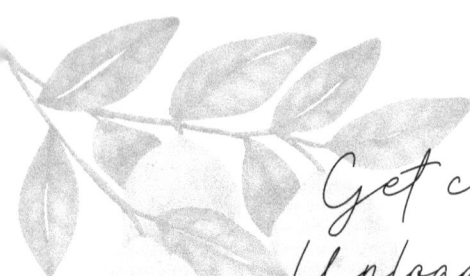

Get connected –
Upload a prayer

There are more than a million words in the English language according to a global language monitoring website. Yet, at times when we want to upload (say) a prayer to our Heavenly Father, we are at a loss of words. It's okay, God is not impressed by your word count.

And don't worry, *our mess of tangled emotions and scattered thoughts are completely known to God before we can so much as vocalize them - Zach Barnhart.*

And when we don't have the words, Jesus speaks to the Father on our behalf (Romans 8:34), in the same way the Holy Spirit helps us in our weakness. We do not know what we ought to pray for, but the Spirit himself intercedes for us through wordless groans (Romans 8:26)

If this is the first time you have prayed to God, it's just like a conversation with him. There is no right or wrong way to pray. He is just thrilled to hear from you.

You can pray from your heart aloud, or silently in a quiet place.

And if you'd like some extra help, I have added some prayers for you. xx

Prayer of healing

Heavenly Father,

Thank you for my life. That I am so privileged to see and hear and smell and taste the work of Your hands.

I come before you today with a heart burdened by illness.

You are the great healer, and I place my trust in Your loving hands. Grant me strength to endure this trial and courage to face each day. Pour out Your healing grace upon my body, mind, and spirit.

And if healing is not according to Your will, equip me and my loved ones with strength, clarity, and discernment. And I pray that You will grant us all Your peace, which surpasses all understanding, to fill our hearts as I endure the days of my Ménière's disease.

In the midst of my weakness, be my strength. I surrender myself to Your care, trusting that Your love will sustain me.

In Jesus' name, I pray,
Amen

Prayer of Thanks

Dear Lord,

I am overwhelmed with the honour that I can come before you and speak to You. Not only do I communicate with You, but You always listen and guide me on the right path.

Thank You for always being there for me, whether I realize it or not. Your love washes over me daily, hourly, and moment-by-moment. I am so fortunate to have you walking with me and loving me, for Your goodness knows no bounds. I am overwhelmed with your goodness and love for me, and for the unceasing love you have shown me throughout my life. You've loved me when I haven't deserved it.

I am so thankful that you accept my prayers and despite all of my failings, you still look upon my love with joy and acceptance. Thank you for being so good to me. Thank you for who You are!

You truly are an amazing God!

In Jesus' name I pray,
Amen

Prayer of Belief

Heavenly Father,

I come to You in the Name of Jesus. Your Word says, "Whosoever shall call on the name of the Lord shall be saved" (Acts 2:21).

I am calling on You. I pray and ask Jesus to come into my heart and be Lord over my life according to Romans 10:9-10. "If thou shalt confess with thy mouth the Lord Jesus, and shalt believe in thine heart that God hath raised him from the dead, thou shalt be saved."

I do that now. I confess that Jesus is Lord, and I believe in my heart that God raised Him from the dead.

Thank you for giving me the gift of eternal life.

I pray this in the name of Jesus,
Amen

Dear Me,

Philippians 4:13

"I can do *all things* through *Christ* who *strengthens me*."

Love, Me

Dear Me,

2 Timothy 1:7

"For God has not given us a
spirit of fear,
but of *power*
and of *love*
and of a *sound mind.*"

Love, Me

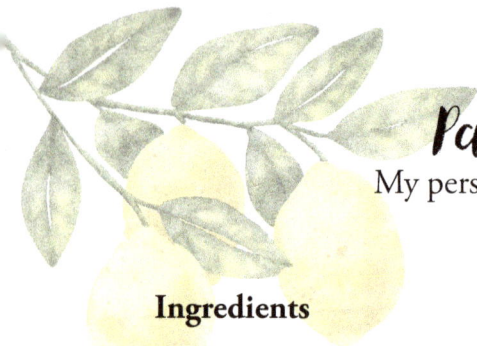

Pavlova
My personal favourite!

Ingredients

4 eggs whites
1 cup caster sugar
1 teaspoon vinegar
1 tablespoon of cornflour
LEMONS for the table decoration!

Directions

Set the oven to 120⁰ C / 248⁰ F

1. Mix the 4 egg whites in a bowl with an electric mixer until stiff peaks form.

2. Add the caster sugar gradually, in small batches, until it is dissolved each time.

3. Add 1 teaspoon of vinegar and 1 tablespoon of cornflour and mix slowly for about ten seconds.

4. On a baking tray, place some baking paper, and sprinkle it with cornflour, to stop the pavlova from sticking to the paper. Then pile on the pavlova mix, keeping it high in a mound (do not spread it out thinly on the baking tray).

5. Bake in the oven for and hour and fifteen minutes. At the end of this time, turn off the oven, but leave the

pavlova in the oven with the door slightly ajar, to let the pavlova cool.

6. When the Pavlova is cool, transfer to a serving plate and decorate with cream and fruits of your choice. I usually add:

- banana
- kiwi fruit
- strawberries
- blueberries
- passionfruit
- raspberries
- mango

7. Eat and enjoy.

Notes (thoughts, photos, tweaks to recipe)

Ménière's Disease Resources

Ménière's Research Australia   Ménière's Society UK
Ménière's.org UK   Vestibular.org   VEDA

Ménière's Journal to track symptoms and find triggers and patterns

Fiction with Ménière's characters,   Dear Ménière's - Letters & Art
or about Ménière's

For kids and adults   Cochlear
Implant Journey

All books can be purchased at online bookstores, or ask your library to order in a copy. Profits from book sales are donated to Ménière's research to help reach that cure or effective treatments for everyone.

About The Author

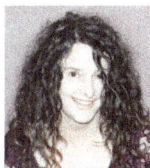

Julieann was diagnosed with Ménière's in 1995. In 2020 she received a cochlear implant. She is the author of a bestselling novel with a **Ménière's character**, *The Colour of Broken*, twice longlisted to be made into a movie. She wrote the sequel - *All the Colours Above* - due to reader requests. She is the author of the *Daily Ménière's Journal*, and *It Will Change Your Life - a cochlear implant journey*. *Vanilla Swirl* and *Blueberry Swirl* are picture books written for children who have a parent who is unwell. In 2023, Julieann released a middle school chapter book called *The Adventures of Captain Vertigo ... and Fart Man* (adults love it too!), and spear-headed *Dear Ménière's – Letters and Art* – a global Ménière's project by people living with Ménière's disease. She is currently working on her 9th novel. She donates 100% of profits from the sales of her Ménière's books (pictured) to research to help find a cure. Julieann is a *Ménière's Research Australia Ambassador*, and also a secondary teacher, artist, chocoholic, tea ninja, paper cut survivor, and tries not to scare off her cat with her terrible cello playing.

julieannwallaceauthor.com
Blog – My Shadow – Ménière's (wordpress.com)
Instagram: @myshadow_menieres
Instagram: @julieann_wallace_author

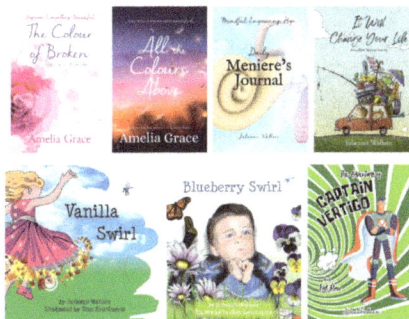

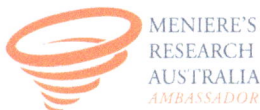

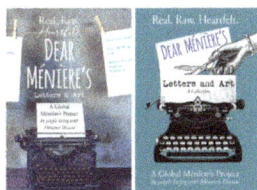

Milton Keynes UK
Ingram Content Group UK Ltd.
UKHW051103190224
438087UK00006B/83

9 780645 158199